Anna Richardson's SUMMER BODY BLITZ DIET

D0480971

700039280865

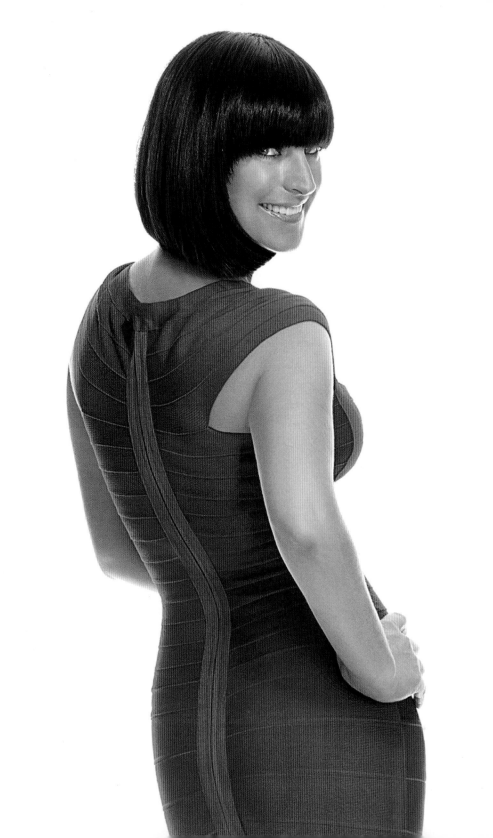

Anna Richardson's
SUMMER
BODY
BLITZ
DIET

Recipes by Justine Pattison

Text © Anna Richardson 2010, 2011
Recipes © Justine Pattison 2010, 2011

The right of Anna Richardson to be identified as the author of the text of this work has been
asserted by her in accordance with the Copyright, Designs and Patents Act 1988.

The right of Justine Pattison to be identified as the author of the recipes of this work has been
asserted by her in accordance with the Copyright, Designs and Patents Act 1988.

First published in paperback in Great Britain in 2010 by Weidenfeld & Nicolson.
This edition first published in Great Britain in 2011 by Weidenfeld & Nicolson, an imprint of the
Orion Publishing Group Ltd, Orion House, 5 Upper St Martin's Lane, London WC2H 9EA.
An Hachette UK Company

1 3 5 7 9 10 8 6 4 2

All rights reserved. Apart from any use permitted under UK copyright law, this publication may only be repro-
duced, stored or transmitted, in any form, or by any means, with prior permission in writing of the publishers
or, in the case of reprographic production, in accordance with the terms of licences issued by the Copyright
Licensing Agency.

A CIP catalogue record for this book is available from the British Library.

ISBN: 978 0 297 86556 8

Photography by Karen Thomas
Location Photography by Chris Gloag
Prop Styling by Liz Belton
Additional styling by Justine Pattison
Thanks to Kitchen Aid, Meyer, Mermaid and Magimix

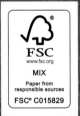

FSC
www.fsc.org
MIX
Paper from
responsible sources
FSC® C015829

Every effort has been made to fulfil requirements with regard to reproducing copyright material. The author
and publisher will be glad to rectify any omissions at the earliest opportunity. Every effort has been made
to ensure that the information in this book is accurate. The information in this book will be relevant to the
majority of people but may not be applicable in each individual case so it is advised that professional
medical advice is obtained for specific information on personal health matters. Neither the publisher nor
the authors accept any legal responsibility for any personal injury or other damage or loss arising from
the use or misuse of the information and advice in this book

Printed and bound in Italy

ADDITIONAL PICTURE CREDITS:
P2 © Nick Holt; P6 © Ray Burmiston; PP26–27 © Momoko Takeda/Getty Images; P29 © Still Images/Getty
Images; P31 © Creative Crop/Getty Images;PP40–41 © Siede Preis/Getty Images; P44 © Peter Dazeley/Getty
Images; P55 © Trine Thorsen/Getty Images

Contents

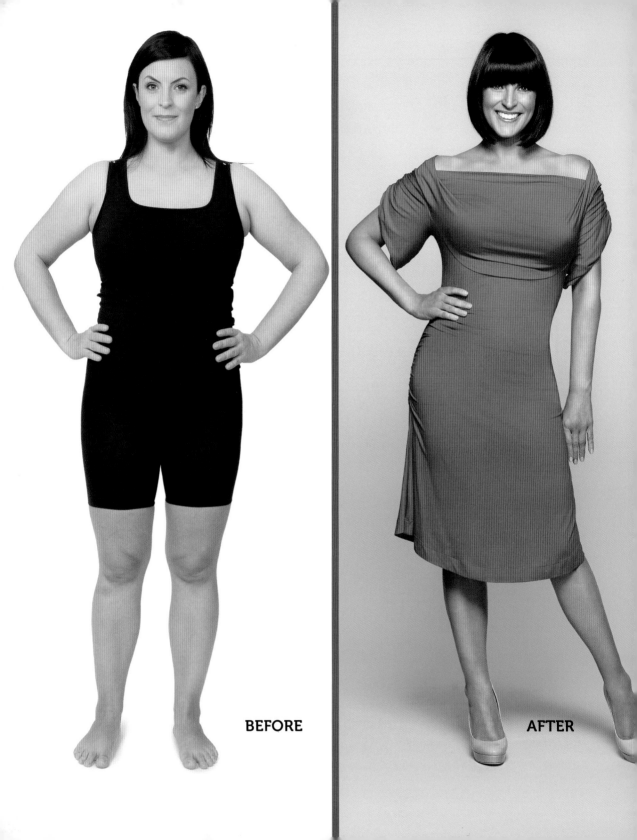

BEFORE

AFTER

My Story

I have a confession to make. I'm sitting here with a Chinese takeaway menu in one hand – and two peppers and a courgette in the other. Weighing up the options. I've fixated on the prawn crackers and crispy fried duck on the menu in my left hand. Mmmmmm.

Ooh…what I wouldn't give to crack open a bottle of beer and pig out on mountains of fried rice whilst slobbing in front of the telly. But then a picture of a little girl on the table catches my eye, and my world comes crashing in. It's a photo of me, just 10 years old, clutching armfuls of biscuits, pop and sweets on her way back to her bedroom to comfort eat because she was so unhappy. And that's it – my fate is sealed. It's taken me no time at all to weigh up my options about what to eat today…because 'weighing up' is what it's all about.

I've discovered a weight loss programme that works; I've lost two stone and I never, ever want to be that fat girl again.

Where Did It All Go Wrong?

So here are the facts. I'm 38 years old; 5 feet 5 inches tall; 9st 7lbs; and a size 10–12. I'm a fat girl struggling to be in a slim body. I'm greedy, lazy and I absolutely love, no, adore food.

Almost to the point of obsession. I'm like Glenn Close in *Fatal Attraction*, never taking no for an answer when I pass the biscuit tin. Like a typical addict, give me just one bite and I'll have to consume the lot. And even though my tummy is saying 'Enough already!' my brain is giving an evil panto laugh and screaming 'Gimme more, more, more!' Nutritionists, hypnotists and doctors have all asked me what my particular food weakness is – Chocolate? Crisps? Bread? And I answer truthfully, no, it's not chocolate or crisps, or bread. It's **EVERYTHING**. And I know exactly how it all started…

One morning, when I was four years old, I woke up to discover my mother had disappeared. Frantic and tearful, I desperately searched the house until my dad explained that mum had been rushed to hospital. Pregnant with my little brother Ben, she was suffering with 'placenta previa' and would have to spend the next two months in a hospital bed. This was most likely the first time my poor dad had ever had to look after his kids alone…and it showed. Never was the phrase 'comfort eating' more relevant than now. Every night – and for the following 56 days – my dad fed me chips from the local chip shop. Fish and chips; beans and chips; sausage and chips; fish fingers and chips; scampi and chips…and gallons of fizzy pop. And even though I laugh whenever my family remembers this, I'm still shocked when my mum tells me that for the next eight weeks I refused to utter a word to her.

I'm about four here and already getting a bit chubby. Who looks more unhappy – me or the donkey??

This is me aged 10. I was very sporty as a kid, but also had a gold medal in overeating.

This is Grandma, my brother Mark, me (aged three and a half), and my mum who's pregnant with my little brother. All was right in my world and I'm a happy, carefree kid.

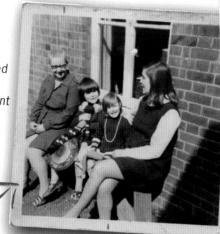

This is me aged 11 and a new girl at boarding school. I was so homesick I used to go to the tuck shop as often as I could to buy food for comfort.

Instead, I would march onto the ward – getting fatter by the day – wash my hands at the corner sink and sing **'Yummy, yummy, yummy there's room in my tummy for some more...for some MORE!'** What I was being starved of in terms of attention, I more than made up for in appetite. And so I became greedy. Greedy for love. And I learned that the more food I could cram into my tummy, the better I would feel about being the little girl who was terrified that her mum had abandoned her.

The pattern was set for good. And for the subsequent 35 years of my life, I have always – always – struggled with my weight. Growing up, I was the fat kid who was made to stand in goal on the hockey pitch. The kid who couldn't run fast because her legs were too heavy. So what would I do? Conduct regular mid-night raids on the kitchens of my boarding school and stockpile biscuits and crisps as though there was a war on. As a young teenager, I was the tubby girl nobody fancied in jumbo cords and a tank top. And at University I reached maximum density through heartbreak and plenty of 12-inch pizzas. Even though I blossomed, became more self-assured and even managed to bag a boyfriend or two, my one true love remained my tummy. It was me, a pie, and my 34-inch stretch elastic jeans. And nothing was going to come between us.

The Good, the Bad and the Downright Dangerous

Of course, there comes a point for every gal when she looks in the mirror, spots the dimples on her bum, the stretch marks on her thighs and the bingo wings wobbling under the t-shirt and she thinks 'Hmmmm…maybe I should go on a diet?'

I've done a quick hand count and I reckon I've tried at least 20 diets over the years, with varying degrees of success. I've bought the cookbooks, supplements, and replacement shakes. The CDs, food blenders and weighing scales. And I've spent a fortune on hope. I would skip intros like this, ignore the chapters on vitamins and nutrition and instead seize upon the holy grail…THE DIET. 'Make me thin!' I would scream at the pages, obsessively calorie counting for three days until I lost interest and fell face forward into a bucket of Maltesers. So I would yo-yo up and down in weight by a stone or two, reserving one side of my wardrobe for fat days and the other for well…fat days.

As a last resort, I kamikazed headlong into total denial and convinced myself that actually, I was really rather slim and that my support pants and sports bra were just for a bit of added contouring on a clearly perfect body.

AND THEN TWO EVENTS IN 2007 CHANGED EVERYTHING…

The first was a shopping experience in Selfridges that left me in tears. Convinced that I was Angelina Jolie's body double (albeit in a pair of Spanx and a G-cup bra) I wandered into the designer dress area to try my luck at finding a figure-hugging gown that would make people weep with envy. Delighted, I found a fabulous size-14 dress by a famous Italian designer renowned for making the best of a woman's curves. Seams splitting, zip straining, bust heaving, I crammed my flesh into the dress and burst forth from the fitting room like an exploding pod. The size-zero assistant looked at me, appalled. 'What do you think?' I beamed. 'My dear...' she replied. 'I tell you this for your own good, and please don't take offence. You need to lose a lot of weight before you can wear a dress like this. You're a nice girl and you're too young to have let yourself go. Go on a diet. Lose that fat. Then come back and see me, because I will make you look fabulous.' I was literally gobsmacked. Cursing her, I struggled out of the dress, flounced out of the store and let the tears roll down my cheeks all the way home.

Two weeks later, I received a call from Channel 4 offering me a job on their new diet series *Supersize v Superskinny*. I was to road test extreme diet regimes and report the truth about weight loss back to the nation. It proved to be a series that would change my life.

On day one of filming, I stepped onto the scales for the first time in seven years and was faced with the shocking fact that I now weighed over 11 stone 7lbs, the heaviest I had ever been in my life. The truth was finally out there, and it hit me straight between the eyes. For the next two months, I tried every crazy regime going to banish that bulge. I ate 40 apples over four days; had surgery on my bingo wings that left my blood pressure dangerously low; tried drinking just maple syrup and water, and even swallowed diet pills. None of them worked. Finally, I hit upon the greatest diet secret the world has ever known.

EAT LESS. MOVE MORE.

Now I manage my addiction to food – and have slimmed down to a healthy 9 stone 7lbs. I'm now two stone lighter, a size 10–12, and happier with my body than I have been for years. I'll never be Angelina Jolie. I'll never be a size zero. But I **CAN** make the best of what nature gave me, and look great.

It's Really Not Rocket Science

Weight loss really isn't rocket science. And I want to break that spell right here, right now.

So I'm sticking two fingers up to the diet industry with a quick and easy **'body blitz'** meal plan that really works. My plan. Based on five simple rules, it's perfect for anyone who wants to bust their gut in as painless a way as possible. It's been tried and tested by ordinary people, is a doddle to follow and guarantees up to a 7lb weight loss with the minimum of fuss in just 14 days. The two-week diet is based on nutritionally balanced, delicious meal ideas and snacks, with no weighing, measuring or counting points. As long as you follow the rules, the pounds – and inches – will simply melt away.

I'm not going to lie to you. It's not revolutionary. But it is common sense. And it works!

Most of you probably don't know this, but a few years ago I co-created the hit TV series *You Are What You Eat,* presented by Gillian McKeith on Channel 4.

I met a brilliant woman on that show called Justine Pattison who writes fantastic recipes and has a passion for making losing weight easy. We have stayed friends, and she was the first person I went to for help when I decided to write this book. Together, we've created something we truly believe in.

Between us, Justine and I have lost over six stone. We know how it feels to be fat. We understand the pain of failure. And we also revel in the joy of slimming success.

So I can promise you that every single recipe Justine has created has been tried and tested. From our own experience we know that the key to successful weight loss is simple recipes that include easily sourced ingredients, have short preparation and cooking times and taste great too!

And finally, I can promise you that if you follow the rules, you **WILL** lose weight, keep it off...and you'll **LOVE IT.**

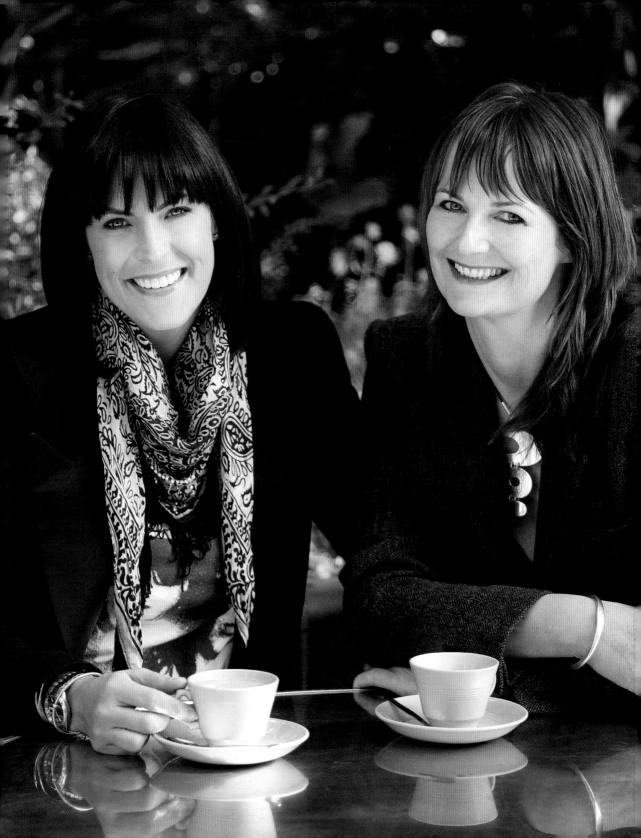

The Rules

So where did we get the idea from for **The Rules**? After all, I'm not a nutritionist, I'm not a doctor, I'm not a dietician. But I **AM** an expert dieter, and **The Rules** are based on knowledge I've picked up along the way from health professionals I've met both here in the UK and in the US. I've found what works for ME...and turned that hard-earned experience into a successful eating plan.

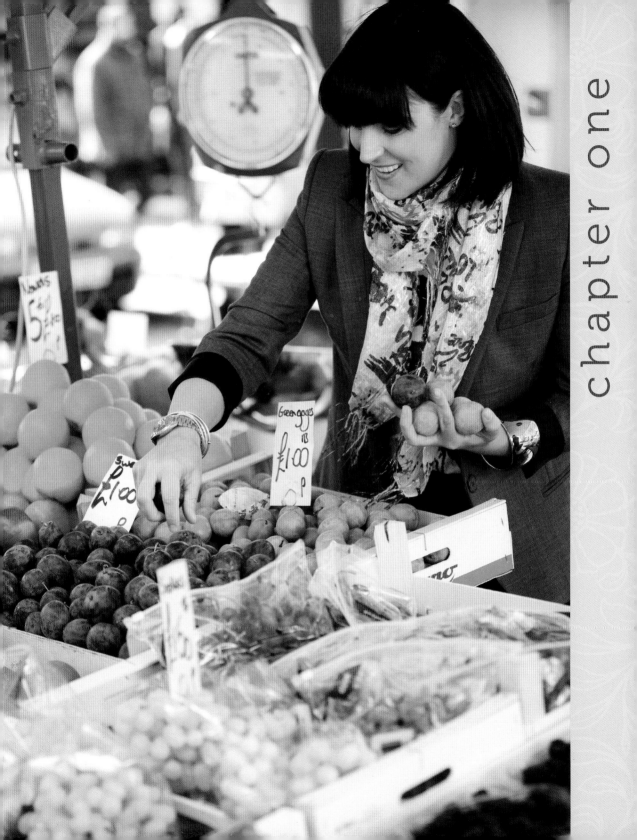

I sat and thought long and hard about what works for me, and I came up with three conclusions. I like to be told WHAT to eat; WHEN to eat it; and that I WILL lose weight if I stick with it. Simple and straightforward. I also want to know that I won't starve, and that the eating plan is sustainable.

So, with **The Rules** I can promise all of the above. It's not rocket science. Just a healthy way to eat and lose the flab in 14 days.

1 NO WHEAT

2 NO DAIRY

3 NO SUGAR

4 NO CARBS (after 6pm)

5 NO ALCOHOL

(6) If you can't manage this for just 14 days then you're NOT ready to diet!

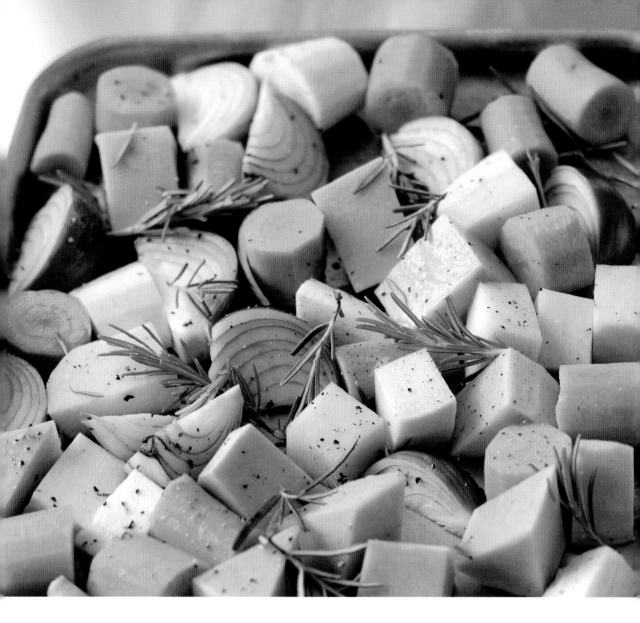

Now, I know what you're thinking. Go on, admit it, you're thinking 'OK, then what the hell CAN I eat?!' If you look at **The Rules** more closely, you'll realise that all I'm asking you to do is eat in a healthy way. In other words no cakes; no cheesy things; no sweets; no booze; and no heavy scoffing after 6pm. So how hard can it really be? It's easy. And I'll hold your hand all the way through.

RULE 1
No Wheat

There's no doubt about it, wheat causes many of us to bloat. The feeling that your waistband is far too tight after you've scoffed a bowl of spaghetti is an all too familiar sensation, isn't it? So, if your belly is making a comfortable pair of elasticated slacks look like an attractive option then it's time to go wheat-free for two weeks and see the difference. You'll not only lose inches around your tummy, but you'll feel heaps better too.

Why cut out wheat?

So why is this rule at the top of my list? You may think I'm going to tell you that wheat is the devil's work designed to line your gut with glue until your waistline begs for mercy. Or maybe that wheat is a carbohydrate that once eaten will suddenly send your insulin levels sky high and lead to the inevitable blood sugar crash. Or something.

Actually, my reasoning is far more straightforward. Foods containing wheat MAKE ME FAT. Have you noticed how once you start with something wheatie, you just can't stop? Bread at the beginning of your meal madam? I rest my case... My tummy always seems to bloat after I've tucked into a couple of slices of toast for breakfast, a sandwich at lunchtime and a big bowl of pasta at night . Even an innocent crumpet will make me look three months pregnant. People have congratulated me on my 'bloom' before now. Little did they know it was just a crusty cob.

I'm no nutritionist, so I don't know why this should be. And, like most people, I definitely don't have an allergy or an intolerance to wheat (oh yes, I've even been tested!). What I do know, however, is that wheat makes me feel uncomfortably full and by cutting it out, I can lose inches around my middle without even trying.

The best thing is that by avoiding wheat, you will automatically cut out a whole load of rubbish from your diet that is just too tempting otherwise.

HERE ARE A FEW OF THE FOODS YOU WON'T BE EATING. JUST SAY **NO** TO THE FOLLOWING FOR THE NEXT TWO WEEKS – AND SEE HOW MUCH BETTER YOU FEEL:

- Batter
- Biscuits
- Bread (except rye bread)
- Breaded fish or scampi
- Buns
- Cakes
- Chicken nuggets
- Couscous
- Cookies
- Crackers

- Croissants
- Crumpets
- Egg noodles
- Garlic bread
- Melba toast
- Muffins
- Packet sauce mixes
- Pasta
- Pastry
- Pies

- Pizza
- Rolls
- Sausages
- Stuffing mixes
- Wheat breakfast cereals, such as Weetabix and Special K
- Wheat flour (plain, self-raising flour, bread flour)
- Yorkshire puddings

What about gluten-free products?

Nice try. And I wouldn't blame you for asking. Gluten-free products are usually completely wheat-free. So what could be better than following my rules, but still tucking into a nice bowl of gluten-free pasta for lunch, and then another and then another?

The problem is, the closer to traditional products these breads, pastas, cakes and biscuits taste, the more you are likely to eat. After all, gluten-free cakes and biscuits are still high in fat and sugar. And the breads and pastas are now so good that they're very easy to overeat. You will lose weight more effectively if you just **AVOID** these foods. Cutting out wheat does NOT mean your life is going to fall apart.

How to avoid wheat

My advice is to look at the ingredients list very carefully before you buy. It will make a huge difference to your weight loss.

● Wheat can be found in foods like bread, croissants, cakes, biscuits, crumpets, rolls and muffins, as well as pasta, pizzas, Yorkshire puddings, pancakes and wraps.

● Wheat is the main ingredient in many breakfast cereals such as **Weetabix, Shredded Wheat, Shreddies, All Bran, Bran Flakes** and those multigrain ones that crop up everywhere. Even muesli contains wheat flakes much of the time.

● You might think you are safe with meat and fish, but pies are a definite no-no because of the pastry; stuffings contain breadcrumbs and sausages are usually blended with wheat rusk. Fish fingers are coated in breadcrumbs and battered fish is enveloped in wheat flour batter.

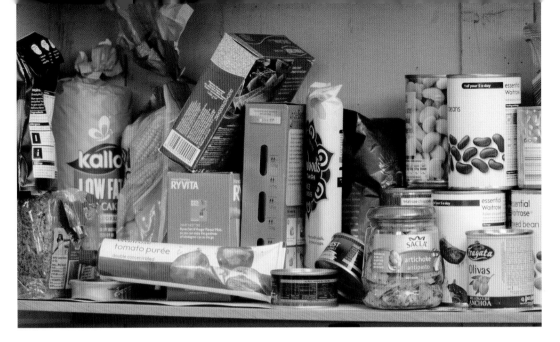

OK...so what CAN I eat?

The list of no-nos will look pretty scary to some of you. But cutting out wheat doesn't mean your life is going to fall apart. Don't panic!

So to fill the gap left by bread and pasta, you'll be able to enjoy foods made with oats, maize (sweetcorn), pulses, rye and rice. Honestly, with these foods to hand there'll be no need to feel hungry. And soon, you'll be saying 'Bread? What bread?'

HERE ARE SOME OF THE FOODS YOU CAN EAT:

- Barley couscous
- Borlotti beans
- Butter beans
- Chickpeas
- Corn cakes

- Kidney beans
- Lentils
- Oatmeal
- Porridge oats
- Rice cakes
- Rice noodles

- Rice – any kind including basmati, jasmine, long grain, camargue red, sushi, paella and risotto
- Rye bread
- Rye crispbread

RULE 2
No Dairy

The no dairy rule is a really tough one for me because I love milk. I'm the sort of classy girl who can drink gallons of the stuff straight from the carton – gross, I know – but hey, who's watching? I used to ram my fridge with loads of different cheeses and no cream cracker would be the same without an inch of butter. I can pack in yogurts two at a time and I'm a sucker for a cream sauce. Hello, my name is Anna and I'm a milkaholic.

You see, as I've said before, I'm greedy. Give me an inch and I'll take the whole milky mile. And let's face it, cheese, cream, milk and yogurts are very, very tasty. And very, very fattening. I finally had to admit to myself that the only way for me to cut down on dairy is to cut it out all together.

Just say NO

So, for two weeks I want you to just say NO. That's no to foods made with full-fat milk, cheese, cream or yogurt. This includes cottage cheese, cream cheese, crème fraîche and fromage frais. Plus, those little yogurt drinks that are packed with sugar as well as friendly bacteria. I want you to cut them out for the moment. You can't swap cow's milk products for those made with sheep's, goat's or any other animal's milk either. I like your style, but it won't work.

This is not a detox diet, it's common sense. It works because cutting out dairy means you cut calories without even thinking. The fewer calories you consume, the more weight you will lose. It is as simple as that.

Won't I miss it?

When I first tried to cut out dairy, I naturally avoided drinking milk in my tea and coffee too. But experience soon taught me that I simply can't get through the day without two or three cups of tea or coffee, and I certainly can't drink them without milk. I also love a bowl of porridge or muesli in the morning, but can't bear it without milk. This diet is meant to be easy and achievable and you shouldn't feel miserable because you're not allowed to enjoy your morning cuppa.

So, an exception to the no dairy rule is SKIMMED or SEMI-SKIMMED MILK in your tea and coffee and for making breakfasts from the meal plan. I reckon that 300ml/½ pint (roughly a large mugful) is enough for hot drinks and breakfast. You don't have to drink it all, but try not to drink more than the allowance. What's more, the calcium contained in milk is especially brilliant for helping us girls avoid dodgy bones in later life too. Hurrah!

HERE ARE SOME OF THE FOODS YOU CAN EAT:

- **300ml (½pint) skimmed or semi-skimmed milk per day in tea or coffee or on cereal**
- **One large skinny or semi-skimmed cappuccino or latte (as part of your daily milk allowance)**
- **Sunflower or olive oil spreads**
- **Soya milk**
- **Rice milk**

What about my butter?!

It's a no to butter for now, gals. I want you to stay away from dairy as much as possible for the next two weeks. However, a smear of sunflower or olive oil spread is absolutely fine – don't go mad though, you should be able to see the colour of your rye bread underneath it!

RULE 3
No Sugar

This one should come as no surprise really. But it's still an interesting one. Every day we're bombarded with images of high-sugar, high-fat snacks that are SO hard to resist. These foods are massively high in calories and we all know deep down that the more of these refined sugar treats you eat, the fatter you get. But they just taste so damn good. I believe that you can easily get hooked on sugar – and if you've ever driven to a garage at midnight in your pyjamas just to buy a Mars Bar (yes, that's me) you'll know exactly what I mean. So wise up and cut it out.

Sweets for my sugar

I've rewarded myself with sweet things for as long as I can remember. When I was a kid, my dad would buy me bottles of sugary Lucozade and piles of toffees when I was ill as a treat to make me feel better. On our way back from school, my mum would always stop at the newsagent for me and my brothers to pile in and buy stacks of space dust, flying saucers and fizzy cola bottles. It wasn't long before I started to steal money out of my mum's purse and cycle to the local shop to secretly buy midnight snacks. If you're relating to this then you'll understand exactly what I mean about sugar being addictive, and a brilliant way to comfort yourself when you're feeling down. Have you EVER been able to eat just ONE chocolate? Unlikely. Just last year, after a row at work that left me feeling really low, I drove into a supermarket car park, bought a bag of 10 mini doughnuts and ate one after the other until the box was empty. Did I feel better? Yes. For about 10 minutes. And then I berated myself for being greedy, fat and stupid and vowed to go on a diet immediately. Why put yourself through the pain and misery? Refined sugar has no nutritional value or benefit – it's pointless. But the weird thing is, once you cut it out – a bit like a wart on your finger – you won't miss it one bit.

If you're flailing about the house right now in a panic about giving up your treats: relax, calm down. I'm going to include a section on snacks later in the book that should satisfy your cravings and that 4pm sugar hunger. And I promise, once you give up refined sugar for good you'll discover that you just don't want it anyway.

HERE ARE A FEW OF THE FOODS YOU WON'T BE EATING:

- Biscuits
- Cakes
- Cereal bars
- Chocolate
- Golden syrup
- Granulated, caster or brown sugars

- Honey
- Ice creams
- Ice lollies
- Jam
- Lollipops
- Maple syrups

- Sugary breakfast cereals
- Sugary fizzy drinks
- Sweets
- Treacle

A sugary P.S.

It doesn't take a genius to understand that losing weight is about feeling good too, and you're never going to feel brilliant when you're tucking into rubbish. So while you're clearing out your cupboards and chucking away your biscuits, sugar and sweets, do the same with crisps and salty snacks too. They're never going to make you thin, are they?

RULE 4
No Carbs (after 6pm)

This rule is a real winner. It's dead easy to stick to and will make all the difference to your flab. Read any interview with a celebrity and time and time again they'll reveal their secret weight loss weapon – **NO CARBS AFTER SIX**.

No-no carbohydrates include any type of bread, rice, cereal, pasta, potatoes etc. If in doubt, avoid anything remotely stodgy, white or beige. You may feel a few cravings in the early days, but your body will soon get used to it, I promise. Just watch it though, ramming down a massive bowl of chicken risotto at 5.45pm defeats the object.

Don't panic! I know a lot of you like to have a starchy carb meal in the evening but try it this way for just two weeks.

Why? Well, when I follow this rule, I always wake up in the morning feeling that bit lighter and brighter and just a tiny bit pleased with myself for not pigging out the night before. I look forward to my breakfast instead of giving it a miss and find it far easier to stick to my meal plan. And the result? Simple. I sleep better, I lose more weight and I can feel the difference around my middle in days. PUT SIMPLY: don't eat starchy carbs with your evening meal – whatever time you have it.

So what CAN I eat in the evening?

Loads – don't worry. Instead of loading my plate up with pasta, rice or potatoes (like I would do in the past) I now fill it with lean protein like chicken breast, lean meat or fish (and tofu or Quorn for the veggies). Why? Because protein takes longer to digest than carbohydrate so it makes me feel fuller for longer. I also stack my plate with loads of fresh vegetables – the more the merrier as far as I'm concerned. I know that if my plate is at least half filled with vegetables or salad, (yes, I do know that vegetables, like fruit, contain carbohydrate, but it's fine to eat them on this diet) I'm not going to feel hungry at the end of the meal, let alone two hours later.

In case you think there won't be much to enjoy, have a look at the delicious recipes and varied choices in the **14 DAY MEAL PLAN**. There's enough there to keep the most demanding of appetites happy.

Listen to your body

At least a couple of times a week, I'm not really that hungry in the evening. There are loads of reasons why we should eat three proper meals a day, but I also think it's really important just to listen to your appetite.

If you're not hungry, then don't eat much but always eat something. If you find that a large breakfast and a good lunch have left you feeling comfortably full and not fancying dinner, great! Nibble on some fruit or try one of my snack ideas (page 194) instead. If you're feeling a bit peckish later, just choose a couple of the quick fixes. Eat according to your appetite and not because you're bored, tired, lonely, miserable, happy, or whatever and you'll never need to diet again.

RULE 5
No Alcohol

I know, I know, this one is a real bummer. But I wouldn't be including this rule if I didn't think it was absolutely necessary. Like most people, I'm the sort of girl who looks forward to a large glass of white wine at the end of a stressful day and dinner wouldn't be the same without a bottle of red now, would it? For me, G&T is the perfect drink for a night out, but then so is beer, vodka, champagne, tequila and rum. So yes, I do like a drink.

But there's no doubt about it, alcohol is bad news when you're trying to lose weight. It's a LOT of fun I know, but alcohol only means empty calories to you and me. It's rapidly absorbed into the body and quickly leads to weight gain if you over-indulge. It's not called a beer gut for nothing!

Wine glasses are bigger than ever before, so although a traditional glass holds around 125ml of wine, you're more likely to serve yourself 250ml in today's measures. That's double. And three large glasses of wine in a pub are the equivalent to a whole bottle. No wonder you're tripping over the step on your way out.

Just think about it. It's recommended that women consume 1200–1500 calories a day if they're trying to lose weight. Two large glasses of white wine contain around 360 – more or less the same as a healthy lunch – yet offer no nutritional benefit. You'll feel hungrier afterwards than you did before. So is it any surprise that you're finding it hard to get slim? What's more, if you're anything like me, after just one glass all your dieting resolve will fly out of the window and you'll be following your vodka with pie and chips.

Low-calorie drinks – say yes!

Many diets, and definitely those with the word 'detox' somewhere in the title, will tell you to avoid low-calorie drinks like the plague. And I've tried, I really have. But, when it comes down to it, sugar-free drinks help me lose weight.

There's something about the fizziness and flavour of these carbonated drinks that curbs my cravings and stops me feeling hungry. Nutritionists say that often your body tells you it is hungry when in fact you're thirsty. After a glass of something bubbly, I know the difference. I'm not telling you to go mad and drink nothing but sugar-free drinks all day – we all know they're full of sweeteners, but I've found two or three cans or glasses can really help and I really want you to succeed this time.

HERE ARE A FEW DRINKS YOU CAN HAVE:

- Slimline tonic
- Lime and soda
- Diet fizzy drinks
- Well-diluted cordials
- Freshly squeezed juices

- SPICY BLOODY MARY
  – without the vodka

- THE CHEAT'S G&T
  Wipe the rim of a glass with gin, fill it up with lots of ice and lemon and pour over slimline tonic

And finally…

I'm only asking you to cut out alcohol for two weeks. The first couple of days might be tricky, but please get through it without resorting to a crafty snifter. I promise you it will be worth it.

And Another Thing…

All right, so you have the **FIVE RULES** which should be a constant mantra in your head for the next 14 days. **REPEAT AFTER ME:** no wheat, no dairy, no sugar, no carbs after 6pm, no alcohol. Easy. To support you along the way, I've also got **FIVE TOP TIPS** that should really help you when it comes to maximising your dieting success.

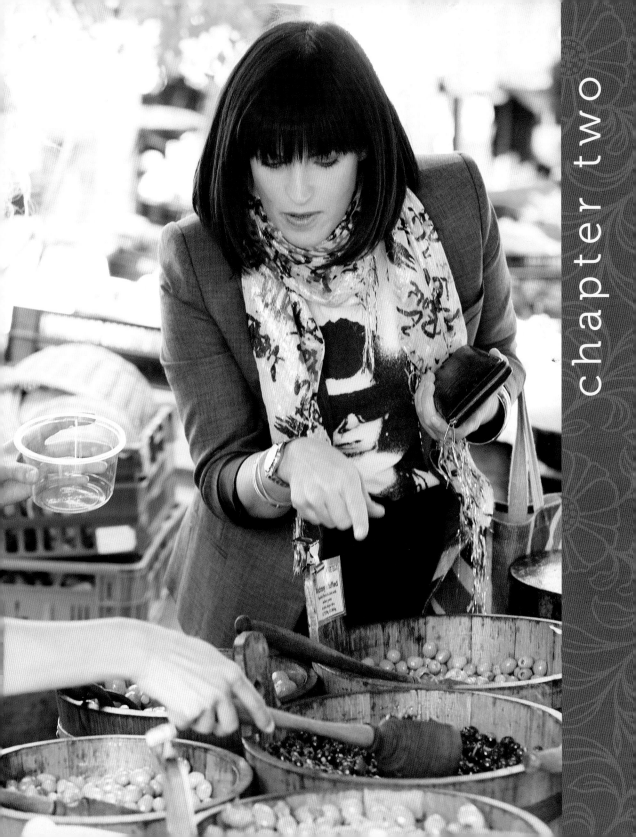

chapter two

MY TOP TIPS to Weight Loss

1. Eat regularly

Yes, yes it's a classic. But that's because it works. When I look back at my porkier years there's a constant theme that rears its ugly head, and it goes something like this: I wake in the morning, late for work, so don't bother eating breakfast; stop at Starbucks and grab a massive latte and muesli bar (all the while kidding myself that 'muesli bar' equals healthy low-fat snack); starve until mid-afternoon then scoff bag of crisps and a load of biscuits; feel guilty, so skip supper – only to cook up three packets of Super Noodles at 10pm before wobbling off to bed like a bloated slug. Any of this sounding familiar?!

So if you want to tackle your tum and fight the flab, do yourself a favour and eat regularly. Try eating proper meals, as eating at regular intervals will stave off the hunger pangs and help make sure your blood-sugar levels remain stable.

2. Eat more fruit and vegetables

I know what you're thinking. Believe me. Is there anything worse than life revolving around vegetables? It all sounds so very dull and, well, worthy. But what you'll find on this plan is that fruit and veg just casually slip into your life like old friends. Old, attractive friends. Ones you want to eat. Lots of. Ones that will make you look, feel and behave in a nicer way. And what better friends are there than that? You should be able to slip a portion of fruit in at breakfast; at least two portions of

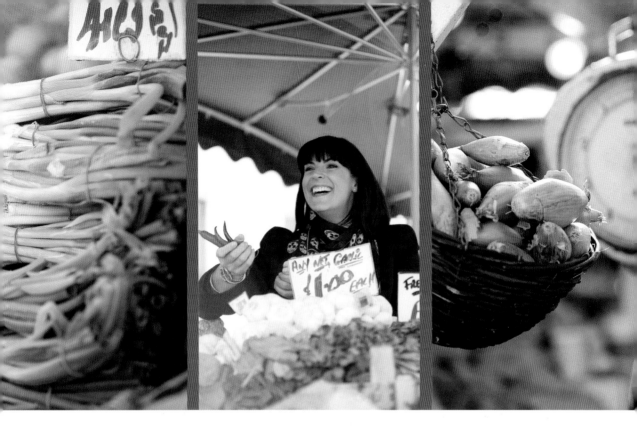

fruit or veg for snacks; definitely a load at lunchtime and the same with your evening meal. Fresh fruit and vegetables fill you up, are delicious and make dieting easy. Not only are they great for weight loss, but your complexion will glow and you'll be treating yourself to a great mix of vitamins to help keep your body in tip top condition.

STOP!

DON'T SCOFF SPUDS. Of course this old fashioned piece of advice automatically excludes all potatoes (and sweet potatoes) – whether they are boiled, baked, roast, mashed, or whatever. And don't forget potatoes that cleverly masquerade as all sorts of tempting snacks. So, all crisps, chips, hula hoops, etc. are out of the question. It's surprising how much easier it is to exclude all potatoes for a couple of weeks than to just have one. And, they're weirdly unappetising once your fortnight is up.

3. Drink plenty of fluids

I'm not going to tell you that you have to down eight glasses of water a day or wander around constantly attached to a bottle of Evian. But there's no doubt about it, drinking plenty of water seems to help me lose weight. I'm not exactly sure why. And I don't know if I go along with the whole 'flushing out toxins' thing. But I do know that if you keep your fluid levels up, your weight will drop.

So, go for two or three cups of tea or coffee, with or without low fat milk plus four or five large tumblers of water a day and you'll not only encourage your body to lose weight but it'll help stop you feeling hungry too. It's a weird thing, when I start to pee a lot, I know I'm starting to shift the pounds too.

4. Don't eat 'diet' food

It's tempting, isn't it? You're on a diet, you go to the supermarket, you want a 'quick fix' to get to size zero overnight. So what do you do? Buy thousands of ready prepared diet meals. You go home, whack one in the microwave, wait for the 'ping' then slob in front of the telly eating a teeny weeny portion of slop.

STOP!

'Diet food' is designed to make money for the food manufacturers and will do you no favours in the long run. It's rammed with additives, artificial flavours, colours and fillers. It's low in fat so it's sure to be high in carbohydrates. Even a tub of low-fat yogurt is likely to contain all sorts of sweeteners, stabilisers and thickeners. Try to eat food as close to its natural state as possible and your body will thank you for it.

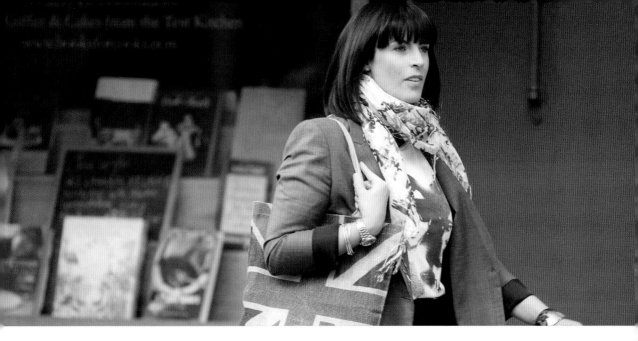

5. Get moving

I'm the last person to put my running shoes on for a rainy jog and the idea of stuffing myself into lycra shorts is enough to make me feel all hot, sweaty, out of breath and in need of a stiff vodka. But, if you want to lose weight and look good at the end of it, exercise is a necessary evil. I don't want to force you down to the local gym, but there's plenty you can do from home to help you get toned and feeling fit. You know what they say: try to find time for at least 30 minutes of exercise five times a week. Even if you break it up into 10-minute slots you'll still reap the rewards. Walk, jog, run up the stairs, vacuum – just move.

Exercise will help you burn calories, increase your metabolic rate and enable you to lose weight faster. Also, the danger of not exercising as you lose weight is that you'll end up pretty flabby. Bingo wings, loose skin around your tummy and a flat, wrinkly bottom. To put it simply, you need muscle structure in place to hang your skin on. It doesn't have to be pounding the treadmill at the gym, it can be dancing or walking the dog. And do you know what? I never thought I'd say this – but it can actually be...FUN.

Before You Begin

The success to any diet is organisation, in fact success in life is down to organisation. If you are clear about what you are doing, why you are doing it and you've prepared yourself every step of the way, the goal just seems to be within sight. And weight loss is exactly the same.

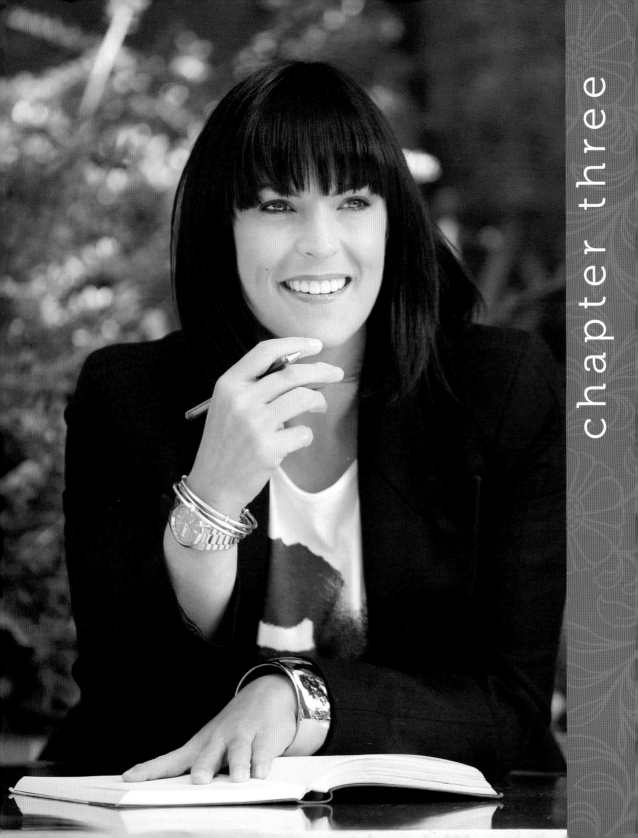

chapter three

What Dress Size Are You...*Really?*

I imagine that the majority of you reading this will be women. Welcome ladies! And if you ARE a girl then you'll know that we all tend to kid ourselves, just a little bit, about our dress size. It's just so much nicer to be able to say 'I'll take that in a size 12 please' rather than 'Have you got a size 16 in the black?' And let's face it, we all compare ourselves to our friends as well, which can be a little depressing if they're naturally very slim (but isn't it great when they still have cellulite? Ha!). So girls...and fellas...it's time to get real about what size we REALLY are and stop squeezing ourselves into clothes that are just too small. Only when you face the truth can you change it.

How to measure yourself

Whenever I've done other diets and they've recommended that you measure yourself I've always thought 'Pah! What a total waste of time. Who cares about measurements, I just want to be thin!' This is all part of self-denial and a weird kind of resistance to facing reality. The reasons I think this is a good idea are:

- It's actually quite interesting to know how your body measures up. Always thought your waist was a trim 28 inches? Get REAL lady, it's 31 inches and the rest!

- You will get IMMENSE satisfaction when you re-measure yourself in two weeks' time and see how many inches you've lost. It's real and you will feel so damn happy.

Once you've done your tape measure torture, make a note of it. It makes sense to match your measurements to the ones given by your favourite clothes shop – you'll find them online if not in store – or check out out the **INDUSTRY STANDARD SIZE CHART** below. Don't freak out, this is just a guide and the total inch loss is what counts. We are all different shapes and sizes.

USA	UK	Europe	Bust	Waist	Hip	Size
2	4-6	32	30-32"	22-23"	30-31"	XS
4	6-8	34	32-33"	23-24"	31-32"	XS-S
6	8-10	36	33-34"	24-25"	32-33"	S
8	10-12	38	34-35"	25-26"	33-34"	S-M
10	12-14	40	35-36"	26-27"	34-35"	M
12	14-16	42	36-37"	27-28"	35-36"	M-L
14	16-18	44	38-39"	28-29"	37-38"	L
16	18-20	46	39-40"	30-31"	38-40"	L-XL
18	20-22	48	41-42"	32-33"	40-42"	XL
20	22-24	50	43-44"	33-34"	41-42"	XL-XXL

That's it, job done. Now you know what dress size you really are. Cheer up – you'll have dropped down a size in just 14 days' time.

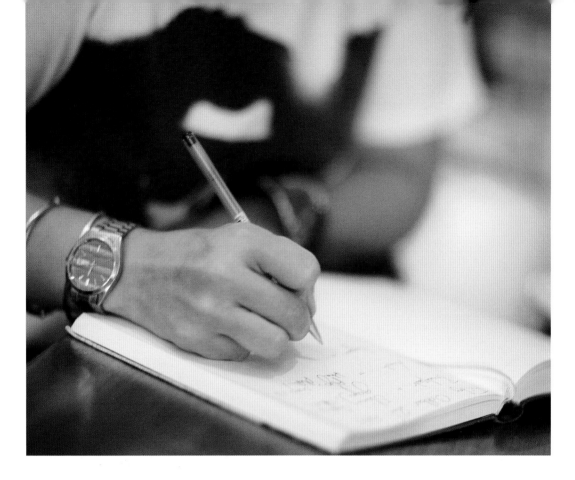

Keep a diet diary and weight loss chart

If there was just one tip that I could ram home to guarantee diet success it would be this one. It was absolutely the secret of my two stone weight loss. I became really quite obsessive about recording the food I ate, what exercise I did and how much I weighed in full Bridget Jones fashion. And I loved every minute of it. Because what you put in, you get back. Just like your body. You take control of your life and reap all the rewards when you start to record your weight dropping.

So go and buy a diary; a big blank book that you can stick photos in; make a spreadsheet on your computer; keep a record on your phone – I don't care how you do it. Just do it.

Take photos

I'm not going to say anything about this other than take a look at the photos below. They were taken six months apart, that's all. And when I had the first one taken I thought I was super slim! Hello?

So, time to get real. Take some photos of your face and body from all angles and stick them on the fridge or in your Diet Diary. You WILL see a difference in two weeks. And you will see a massive difference if you keep going for longer. Believe me, when you look back at your tubby self you'll be amazed.

January

'I've never been one to put weight on my face so it was a shock when I took this photo for my diet diary and could only see a moon face.'

July

'This was taken just six months later and you can see the difference in my face. It motivated me to keep away from the junk.'

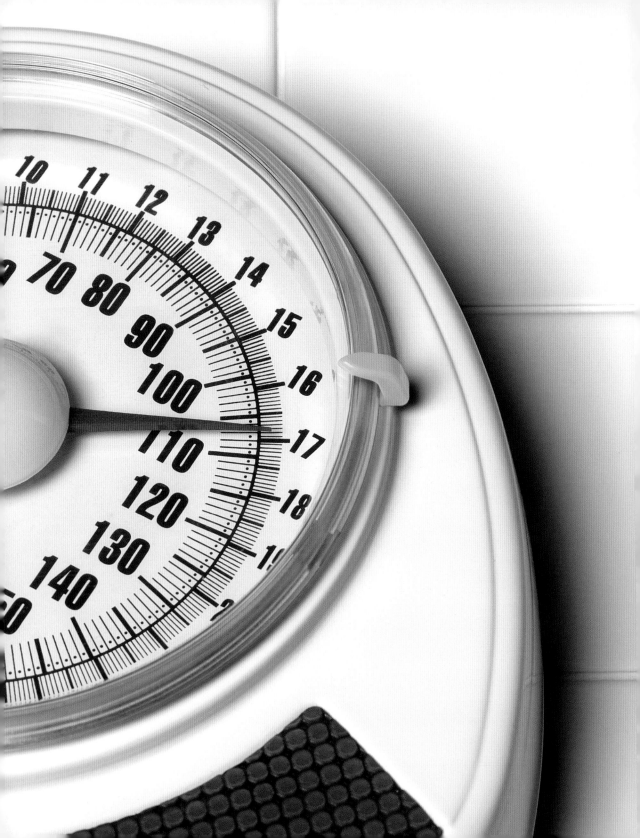

The Importance of Weighing Yourself

This really is my favourite test of all time. I've been a member of various diet clubs on and off for years, and whenever I joined I would give strict instructions to the lady weighing me NOT to tell me what my weight was. I just couldn't face it. So when I started series one of *Supersize v Superskinny* I had to face the truth and agreed to be weighed on camera, even though I hadn't looked at a pair of scales for seven years.

In my head, I was 10 stone and a size 12. When I stepped on the scales, I nearly burst into tears when they tipped in at 11 stone 7lbs. That was it. My house of cards tumbled, and I had to accept that I was a porker who was secretly cutting out the labels of size 16 dresses. And do you know what? It was the best thing that could have happened to me.

Listen, for some of you it might be a painful reality. I do understand, I've been there during my yo–yo dieting. But this is a crucial step towards becoming a slimmer you and keeping the weight off for good.

Now that I've hit a weight that I'm happy with, I still make sure I weigh myself every week just to monitor the flab and stop it creeping up on me!

Once you've got over the shock, record your weight in your Diet Diary. Do it every day, even if your weight stays the same for the first few days.

Getting Started

So, you've decided to go for it. **CONGRATULATIONS!** Maybe you've got a special dress or a favourite pair of jeans you want to fit into in a fortnight, or perhaps you're thinking more long term. Whatever your reason for making the decision to lose weight, **WELL DONE**.

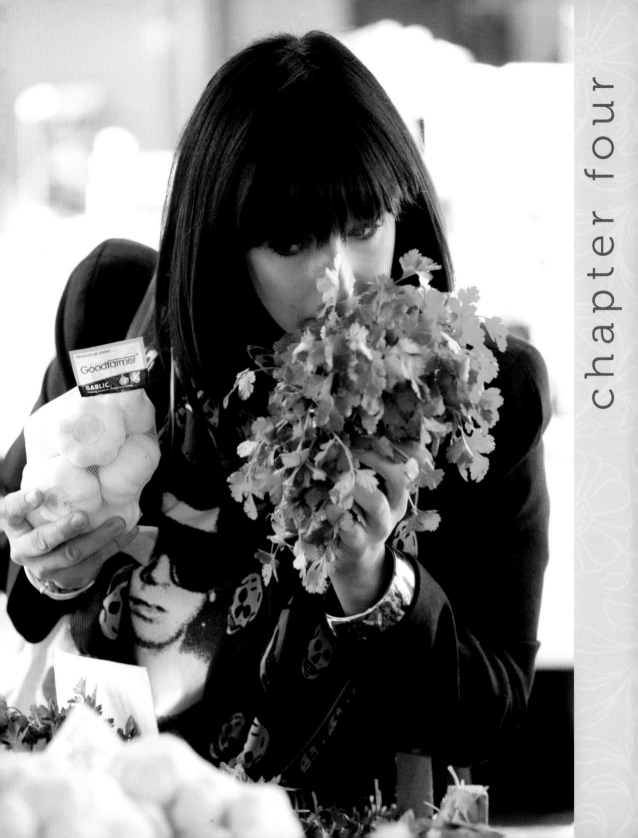

chapter four

The Decision's Made

BUT, and I hate to say it, deciding you want to lose weight is the easy part. What comes next is the tricky bit. And, if you're anything like me, you've been wanting to lose weight for most of your life. So, what's stopping you achieving your dream?

It could be emotional entanglements, a hectic work schedule, boozy social life or a manic family life that puts you at the bottom of the priority list. And sometimes, just sometimes, it's just down to pure laziness. It's true. I know plenty of people who'll eat a couple of chocolate bars for breakfast, grab a large burger and fries at lunchtime and order a takeaway meal in the evening. And guess what? They're all overweight. It's not because they don't know how to cook either, it's because they simply can't be bothered. And if that sounds like you, I understand – believe me – but now is your time to lose weight. You've got to decide, just like I had to decide: either accept that you're going to be unhappy about your weight for the rest of your life or do something about it.

You have to fix the stuff in your life that makes you fat. And you can. It's all about taking control. You are overweight because you've been eating too much of the wrong food. And with the **Summer Body Blitz Diet** you can put that right.

When your eating habits are in check, everything else seems to slot into place. You'll feel more confident and able to cope better with whatever life throws at you. Honest. Imagine a life that doesn't revolve around your relationship with food and the guilt of overeating. It's incredibly liberating.

If you can stick to **The Rules** for the next fortnight, you should be well on your way to the body you've always dreamed of. It might not be perfect, but it's your body and you should look after it. After all, hopefully you're going to be together for a very long time.

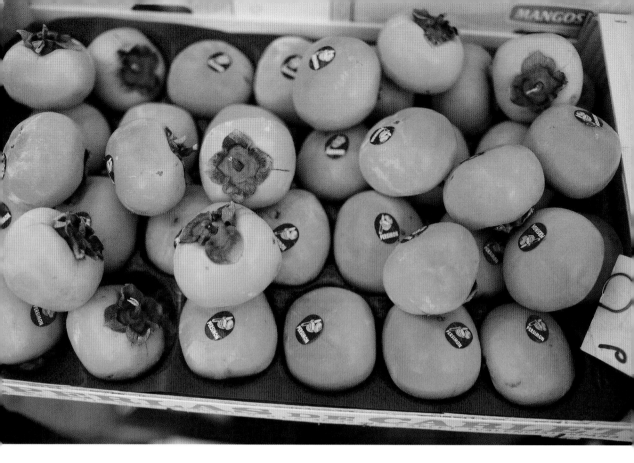

Make It Easy On Yourself

Now you know all **The Rules**, you could stop reading the rest of the book and go off and lose up to 7lbs over the next two weeks. It could be as simple as that. But loads of people, and I'm one of them, like to have something a bit more formal to follow. So, Justine and I have written up a **14 Day Meal Plan** that includes lots of delicious meals and snack ideas. We've kept it dead simple so there's no excuse not to stick to it.

We've also incorporated lots of tips and ideas into the next section to help you along the way. These are all things that have worked really well for me and should be equally as successful for you.

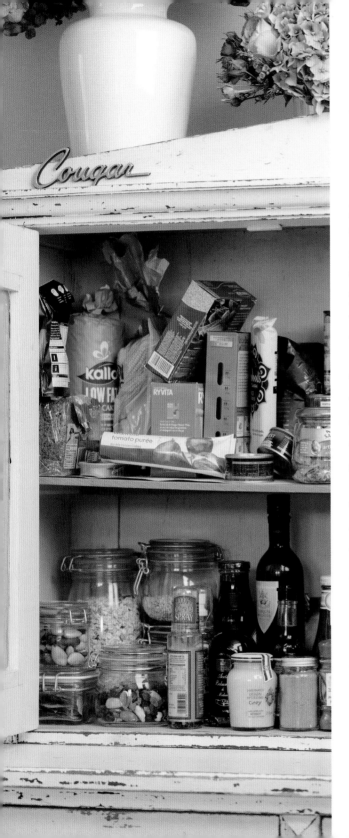

Stocking Up

I know that one of the most important things for weight loss success is to make sure that you are well stocked with all the foods you can eat when you're following the plan. And, that's not just stuff for the fridge, it's about the store cupboard as well.

We've worked out that the key to losing weight is to make the meal ideas as simple as possible, so you won't find any weird ingredients or supplements in our recipes.

Loads of ingredients are bound to be in your cupboards anyway, but if not, they're all easy to get hold of in most supermarkets and even corner stores.

On the opposite page is a list of the store cupboard ingredients that you could need. After all, who wants to drive all the way to a health food store to locate an ingredient you can't pronounce let alone digest?

Store Cupboard Diet Weapons

HERE'S A LIST OF THE **STORE CUPBOARD INGREDIENTS** THAT YOU COULD NEED OVER THE NEXT FORTNIGHT:

• OILS & VINEGARS

Extra virgin olive oil
Mild cooking oil spray
Olive oil
Sunflower oil
Good balsamic vinegar
White wine vinegar

• JARS

Baby capers
Char-grilled artichokes
Char-grilled peppers
Crunchy peanut butter
Dijon mustard
Mango chutney
Medium curry paste
Olives (black and green)
Pickle
Semi-dried (Sun Blush)
tomatoes in oil
Tomato and basil
stir-through pasta sauce
Tomato pasta sauce
Tomato puree
Yeast extract (Marmite)

• SAUCES

Caribbean-style
hot pepper sauce
Dark soy sauce
(Most soy sauce contains small amounts of wheat – don't worry about it. The quantities are so tiny, they're not going to make any difference to your weight loss.)
Hoisin sauce
Hot horseradish sauce
Ketchup
Mayonnaise
Salad cream
Sweet chilli dipping sauce
Worcestershire sauce

• DRY INGREDIENTS

Arborio risotto rice
Basmati rice
Beef, chicken, lamb and
vegetable stock cubes
(Most stock cubes contains small amounts of wheat – don't worry about it. The quantities are so tiny, they're not going to make any difference to your weight loss.)
Corn cakes
Cornflour
Dry rice noodles
Easy cook long grain rice
Jumbo porridge oats
Pearl barley
Popping corn
Puy lentils
Rice cakes
Rye crispbread
Red lentils

• NUTS AND DRIED FRUITS

Almonds (blanched
and flaked)
Dried apricots (no soak)
Hazelnuts
Mixed nuts
Mixed dried fruit

Sweet treats

You'll no doubt notice that some of the sauces listed over the page contain sugar. And yes, I do realise that you're not meant to be eating sugar on the plan. Now, the way I see it is this:

- If there's a way that I can help you succeed, I'm going to suggest it.

- Many sauces do contain sugar, but because you'll be always serving them with lean protein or vegetables, it's very different to eating a chocolate bar, stirring syrup into your porridge or spooning jam on your toast.

So every now and then it's fine for you to add a little ketchup on your plate, drizzle some sweet chilli sauce over your stir-fry or brush your kebabs with a spicy barbecue sauce. I'm certain that by letting the occasional sweet treat into the plan, you'll be more likely to succeed. Just don't go crazy, please.

Herbs and spices

Herbs and spices add lots of flavour and can make a real difference to your cooking without adding calories. Here are the ones we've used for the recipes:

- Black peppercorns
- Cinnamon sticks
- Chinese five spice powder
- Coriander seeds
- Dried chilli flakes
- Dried mint
- Dried mixed herbs
- Dried rosemary

- Dried sage
- Dried thyme
- Flaked sea salt
- Ground cinnamon
- Ground coriander
- Ground cumin
- Hot chilli powder
- Medium curry powder

Cans

Keep cans of these ingredients in the cupboard and you'll be able to make a variety of different dishes.

- **Chopped tomatoes**
- **Mixed beans**
- **Butter beans**
- **Reduced-fat coconut milk**
- **Canned tuna in olive or sunflower oil or water**
- **Cannellini beans**
- **Chickpeas**
- **Red kidney beans**
- **Sweetcorn**

Fruit

Fruit satisfies my sweet tooth and it's healthy in its natural state. Don't avoid fruit, I know some diets tell you not to go near it but what's better for you? A Mars Bar or an apple?! Fruit is easy and there's such a huge choice all year round. I tried a fresh fig the other day and now I'm hooked. It's worth remembering if you eat too much your weight loss will slow down, so keep snack servings to something like one apple, a bunch of grapes, half a punnet of strawberries or one banana.

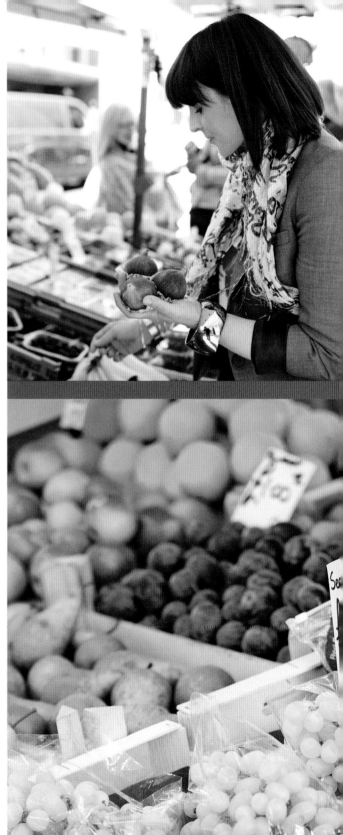

Secret Weapons

Now, there are a few utensils that are going to make following this diet even easier. These are the things that I have in my kitchen to help me prepare the recipes and if you are anything like me, the simpler something is, the more likely I am to do it.

Cooking oil spray

The easiest way to cut calories I know. Most of the major supermarkets now sell these handy little oil dispensers and I love them! They're brilliant because they mist a pan with just enough oil to fry without adding loads of calories.

I always choose the ones with a pump action spray rather than an aerosol, as the oil they use is not adulterated with water or propellants. I have two in my kitchen at all times. I use a mild – almost tasteless – olive oil for frying and an extra virgin olive oil for spraying onto salads. (Drizzle with a little balsamic vinegar and you've got a dressed salad in seconds. Easy.) You only need to press five or six times to mist a large frying pan and then you're ready to start cooking.

If you can't get hold of spray oil to begin with, use a pastry brush or even just kitchen paper lightly dipped in oil and wipe around the pan. Then you'll avoid that fatty, nasty oil slick.

Non-stick frying pan

If you don't already have a decent non-stick pan, then think about investing in one. You'll need to use far less oil in your cooking and the results will be better than ever. And as a completely novice cook, I should know! The best ones are

quite pricy but will last for years –
and think what you'll be saving on
takeaways. The pan should have a
sturdy, flat base and gently sloping
sides. A large one can double up as a
wok if needed, but smaller frying pans
are useful for omelettes and cooking
for one. Choose a pan with a decent
non-stick coating and take care not
to use metal utensils or the non-stick
coating could easily get scratched.

Measuring jug,
scales and spoons

Measuring jugs are really useful
for accurately gauging liquid
ingredients like stock, milk, juice or
water and you can pick them up for
 a couple of quid in many large
supermarkets. They've even got some
good ones in the pound shops. The
recipes in this book don't tend to
call for really exact quantities, but
occasionally a jug is needed. The
same goes for scales and a set of
metric spoon measures. They're not
absolutely necessary but will help
make the recipes even more foolproof.

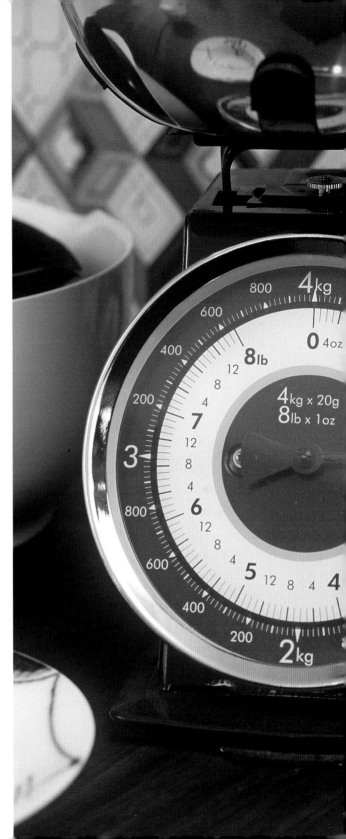

The 14 Day Meal Plan

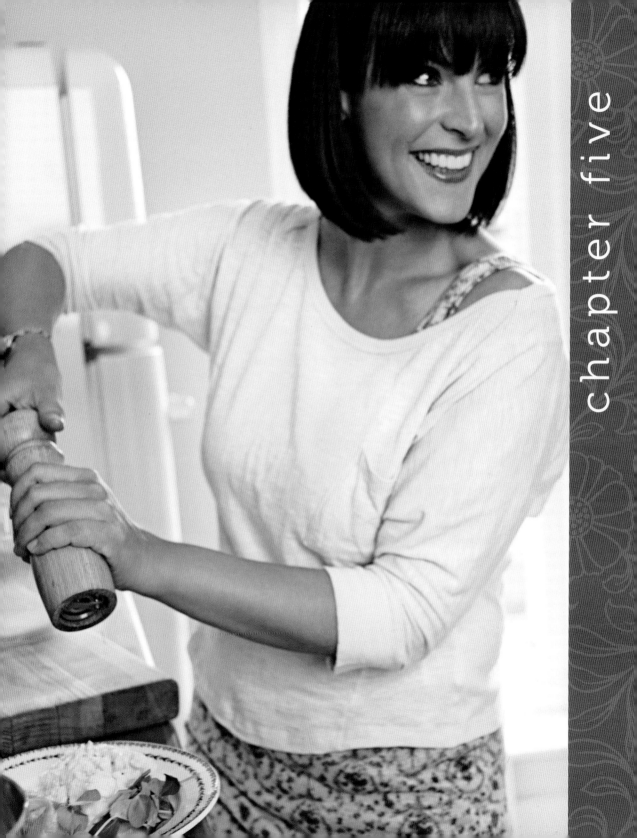

chapter five

The Next Two Weeks

OK, so now you know all the basics, it's time to see what you could be eating over the two weeks on the plan. If you're the sort of person who likes to follow a diet to the letter, we've devised 14 days of meals to keep you right on track. Most of the ideas are dead easy to throw together, but we've also given you loads of really easy recipes to follow, with no complicated methods or weird ingredients. And if I can cook them, anyone can. Believe me.

We've kept it all as basic as possible, including lots of foods that you're probably cooking or eating anyway – just prepared the **Body Blitz** way. If there's something you really hate or can't eat, such as meat, you can simply swap the recipe for something else in the same section of the book.

We're starting you off on a Monday, saving longer recipes for the weekend when you've got a bit more time.

We've also given you a choice of a **Dinner for Two** or **Family Food** each evening. Weekend dishes are designed for more than two, so whether you are cooking for your family or preparing a dinner for friends, there's no need to miss out. If you're feeding a crowd but fancy one of the **Dinners for Two**, just increase the ingredients accordingly. And vice versa. If one of the family meals looks particularly tempting, make it but freeze the leftovers for another time.

Remember this plan is only for two weeks. It really shouldn't be that difficult to stick to. I promise!!

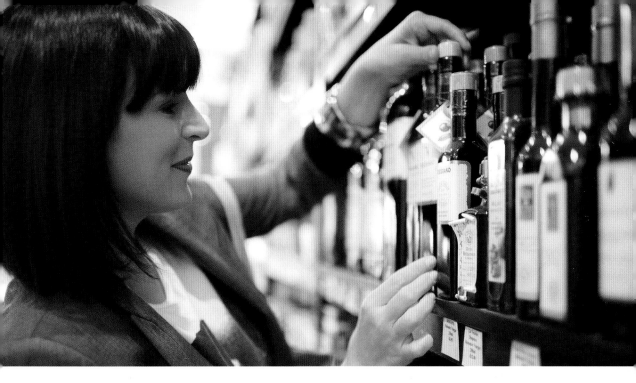

Make it easy

- I've got loads of plastic freezer-proof containers, so I can freeze any food that doesn't get eaten up straight away.

- I like to make some homemade muesli when I can. It makes a convenient and filling breakfast – and it's easy to keep at work. Make a batch of muesli before you start the diet. This will provide you with enough to take you through the two weeks. Store in an airtight container. Easy!

- Whenever I snack on soup, I find that I definitely eat less during my other meals, simply because I feel fuller for longer. You should give it a go. Make at least one vegetable soup to keep you going in the first few days. Eat whenever you fancy it.

- Rye bread will start to go mouldy after a few days in a warm kitchen, so freeze it instead and take a couple of slices out a day. Store crispbreads in airtight containers to prevent them going soft.

Eat plenty of vegetables and salad

- Aim to cover at least half your plate with vegetables. After you've munched your way through a huge pile of greens, there's no way you'll be hungry for hours. And if vegetables aren't really your thing, please do try to give them a go. You'll feel so much better for it.

- Have a variety of vegetables ready in the fridge to serve with your main meals. They'll only take a few minutes to boil – or steam if you prefer. I always have a few carrots, courgettes, green beans and broccoli knocking about, but you can buy packs of ready prepared vegetables or even frozen veg if your food preparation skills aren't up to much. And try not to overcook them. Vegetables that have a little 'bite' taste loads better and retain more vitamins too.

- I'm a huge fan of those packs of ready prepared salad but they can be pricy and go mouldy really quickly, so although I'll buy one or two bags a week, I'll supplement them with baby gem and romaine let-tuces which keep very well in the fridge. Choose the ripest, reddest tomatoes you see – they'll have so much more flavour. Store in the fridge but try to let them stand for at least 30 minutes before serving if you can. They taste a lot better when they're not freezing cold.

- I really like crisp salads with lots of sweet peppers, sliced cucumber, celery and ripe tomatoes, but you could add any other vegetables you fancy: carrot sticks, sliced pickled beetroot or raw mangetout, for example. Just make them as delicious, colourful and as filling as possible.

- It's worth remembering that although fruit, salads and vegetables can be quite expensive, especially in the winter months, you'll be saving pounds overall just by cutting out the junk from your diet.

- Keep a bottle of really good balsamic vinegar to hand and there's no need to worry about complicated dressings either. Just spray your salad with a little olive oil and drizzle with a few drops of balsamic vinegar. Or, make up a quantity of *Body Blitz* dressing and keep in the fridge.

Body Blitz dressing

3tbsp mayonnaise

1tbsp cold water

1tsp freshly squeezed lemon juice

good pinch mixed dried herbs

freshly ground black pepper

Makes 4–6 servings

1. Put the mayonnaise in a small bowl and gradually stir in the water until smooth.

2. Add the herbs and lemon juice. Season with ground black pepper.

3. Cover tightly. The dressing keeps in the fridge for up to 3 days.

A note for vegetarians

You'll see that many of the recipes use meat and fish, but that doesn't mean you can't follow the plan. Simply swap meat dishes for some of the vegetarian alternatives, or use meat substitutes instead.

Quorn or soya mince can be used instead of minced beef in most cases, although you'll need to jig the cooking times accordingly. For the casseroles, like the Lamb Tagine and Beef with Butter Beans, or the curries and rice dishes, you can use Quorn pieces or increase the quantity of vegetables. Firm or marinated tofu is perfect for the stir-fries if you add it towards the end of the cooking time. Make sure you include lots of beans in your diet and snack on nuts as these will both contribute towards your protein intake.

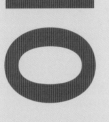

WEEK ONE

MONDAY

BREAKFAST
Homemade muesli
with berries (p75)

LUNCH
Ham and egg with cress (p91)

DINNER
Pan-fried salmon with
stir-fried vegetables (p143)
Or Bolognese with
cheat's spaghetti (p175)
Large lightly dressed salad

TUESDAY

BREAKFAST
Boiled egg and
soldiers (p79)

LUNCH
Chunky vegetable soup (p115)
and Quick Fix platter (p193)

DINNER
Lemony chicken wrapped
in Parma ham (p151)
Freshly cooked vegetables
Or Homemade burgers (p172)
Large lightly dressed salad

Day One

*Get excited. You're about to
go on a guaranteed weight
loss journey! I've already
tried on my favourite jeans
to get a visual estimate on
the 'muffin top' overhang. I
know this will be significantly
better in just two weeks.
Note down your starting
weight and measurements.
Don't faint...*

Day Two

*I've discovered a secret
weapon. Large skinny
cappuccino – that's my milk
allowance gone but it was
worth every sip! Perfect
take-out for car journeys,
boring meetings, or 'between
meals' emergency fill up.
If you're nowhere near a
coffee shop, then buy one
of those granny flasks.
No excuses.*

WEDNESDAY
BREAKFAST
Fruity porridge (p76)
LUNCH
Chunky vegetable soup (p115)
and Quick Fix platter (p193)
DINNER
Peppered steak with
mushrooms (p155)
Freshly cooked vegetables
Or Baked fish with
tomatoes and olives (p163)
Large lightly dressed salad

THURSDAY
BREAKFAST
Homemade muesli
with berries (p75)
LUNCH
Prawn and
avocado salad (p92)
DINNER
Lemon and black
pepper chicken (p158)
Large lightly dressed salad
Or Sticky chicken thighs (p171)
Large lightly dressed salad

Day Three

*I'm a little bit ratty...
I think it may be my body
reacting to the fact I'm no
longer pigging out on bread,
sugar and wine. I'm
sticking with it though,
as I know it's just a
temporary blip.*

Day Four

*My willpower has been tested
to the limit. I've discovered
an escapee mini chocolate
bar in my cupboard. It may
be small, but it's the devil.
Do like the government
recommends with the
flu virus – catch it,
kill it, bin it.*

The Meal Plan

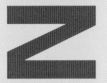
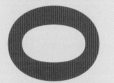
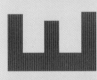

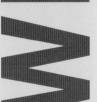

WEEK ONE

FRIDAY

BREAKFAST
Fruity porridge (p76)
LUNCH
Smoked salmon with
watercress and lemon (p92)
DINNER
Quick prawn balti (p140)
Large lightly dressed salad
Zesty fruit salad (p87)
Or Creamy chicken curry (p167)
Large lightly dressed salad

Day Five

Yay! I jumped on the scales
this morning to weigh
myself. I've lost 3lbs in
under five days. It may be
a small step for man but
it's a giant leap for
(wo)mankind. My tummy
definitely looks a little
flatter. This is all the
incentive I need to carry on.

SATURDAY

BREAKFAST
Pan-fried bacon with
mushrooms and tomatoes (p84)
LUNCH
Easy chicken and
mushroom risotto (p99)
DINNER
Tuna Niçoise (p128)
Or Fruity lamb tagine (p185)
Large lightly dressed salad

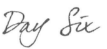

Day Six

I've been invited to
birthday drinks. In theory,
this could be a tricky one
as normally I'd quaff G&T
until I fall over. But no! I feel
rather self-satisfied refusing
all the sugary alcohol, and
can kid myself into thinking
I'm not missing out by
drinking large quantities of
Slimline Tonic with a dash of
lime. Honestly – give it a go.

Anna's Tip

Remember your two snacks a day of either fruit or other nibbles. I've included
lots of ideas in **SNACKS AND DRINKS** (p194).

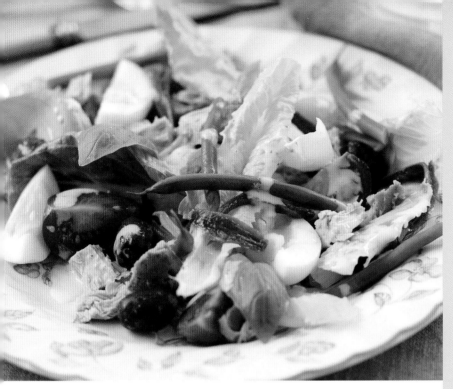

SUNDAY

BREAKFAST

Scrambled egg with smoked salmon and watercress (p80)

LUNCH

Lemon roasted chicken (p168)
Freshly cooked vegetables
Or Spicy bean and vegetable soup (p122)
Slice of rye bread

DINNER

Quick Fix platter (p192)
Large mixed salad

Day Seven

The perfect lazy day. I filled up on a healthy cooked breakfast, then joined friends for a roast lunch. It's easy – just stick to chicken breast and load up on vegetables (no roasties!). After an afternoon walk to pound off the pounds I'm so pleased with myself I don't feel like dinner. Just a few grapes and a cup of tea.

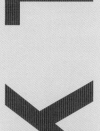

WEEK TWO

MONDAY
BREAKFAST
Homemade muesli
with berries (p75)
LUNCH
Roast chicken with Parma
ham and avocado (p91)
(Make with leftover chicken
from Sunday lunch.)
DINNER
Balsamic salmon (p159)
Large lightly dressed salad
Or Meatballs in
tomato sauce (p180)
Large lightly dressed salad

TUESDAY
BREAKFAST
Homemade muesli
with berries (p75)
LUNCH
Quick Fix platter (p193)
Large mixed salad
DINNER
Sweet chilli beef salad (p130)
Or Gardener's Pie (p179)
Freshly cooked vegetables

Day Eight

OK guys, you're one week in! How are you feeling? By now you should be over any beginner's blips and well into the rhythm of eating properly. Remember, the challenge of every dieter is to stay organised. If you're stressed, disorganised and out of control you'll take your eye off the ball and end up overeating a load of rubbish again. Stay focused.

Day Nine

Oops...I forgot to eat breakfast, I was so busy. A classic dieting error. By mid-morning I'm so hungry I could chew my fingers off. Big mistake. Make sure you have your breakfast every day! It really does help.

WEDNESDAY

BREAKFAST

Scrambled egg on rye bread
with grilled tomatoes (p80)

LUNCH

Tuna with tomatoes and
salad cream (p92)

DINNER

Chicken with chilli
and lime (p158)
Large lightly dressed salad
Or Sausages with
onion gravy (p183)
Freshly cooked vegetables

THURSDAY

BREAKFAST

Fruity porridge (p76)

LUNCH

Quick Fix platter (p193)
Large mixed salad

DINNER

Mexican-style salmon (p139)
Freshly cooked vegetables
Or Lamb Koftas with minty
cucumber salad (p186)

Day Ten

*Are you ready? Take all of
your clothes off. All of them!
And take a long, hard look at
yourself in a full-length mirror
from all angles. Now don't
tell me you haven't shifted a
few pounds! Come on...you're
looking and feeling a little bit
slimmer, aren't you?!*

Day Eleven

*Had a really stressful day
with work today – my
natural reaction would be
to eat a loaf of bread or a
family-size bag of crisps,
for comfort. But no! Instead,
I rummaged around the fridge
and ate a few handfuls of
wafer-thin ham instead.
Job done.*

The Meal Plan

WEEK TWO

FRIDAY

BREAKFAST
Homemade muesli
with berries (p75)

LUNCH
Quick Fix platter (p193)

DINNER
Warm chicken salad (p158)
Or Mini cottage pies with
parsnip and apple mash (p176)
Freshly cooked vegetables

SATURDAY

BREAKFAST
Scrambled egg with smoked
salmon and watercress (p80)

LUNCH
Chilli con carne with rice (p104)

DINNER
Lemony chicken wrapped
in Parma ham (p151)
Freshly cooked vegetables
Or Baked fish with
tomatoes and olives (p163)
Large lightly dressed salad

Anna's Tip

Remember your two snacks a day of either fruit or other nibbles. I've included
lots of ideas in **SNACKS AND DRINKS** (p194).

Day Twelve

*One of the secret
weapons I swear by is
homemade soup. If I eat
a nice big bowl it'll fill
me for hours and stops
me eating rubbish. I got
home from work late
tonight, didn't fancy
cooking, so I just reheated
some vegetable soup
that I'd made at the
weekend.*

Day Thirteen

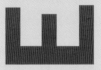

*I woke up today and
noticed that my tummy was
flatter – much flatter. It
put a nice big smile on
my face for the rest of
the day AND my other
half has noticed!*

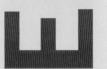

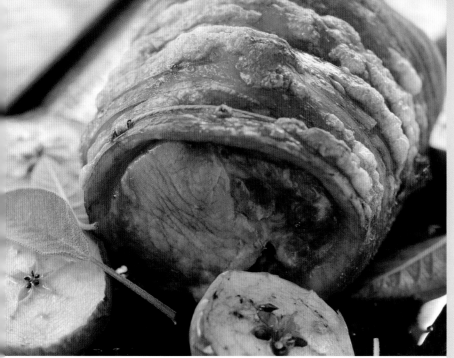

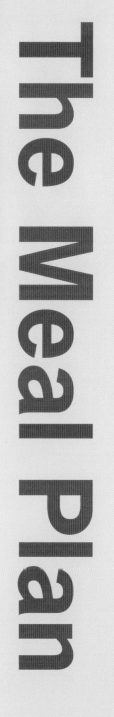

FRIDAY

BREAKFAST

Poached egg with wilted
spinach and grilled tomato (p83)

LUNCH

Roast pork with baked
apples (p182)
Freshly cooked vegetables
Or Gardener's Pie (p179)
Freshly cooked vegetables

DINNER

Quick Fix platter (p193)
Large lightly dressed salad

Day Fourteen

*Congratulations! Fourteen
days of straightforward
healthy eating AND a dress
size less to boot. Admit it…it
really wasn't that bad after all,
was it? You should be feeling
slimmer and thinking slimmer.
And if you're like me, then
you'll be feeling so pleased
with your weight loss that you
may just want to keep it up for
a bit longer. You go for it! And
well done.*

The Recipes

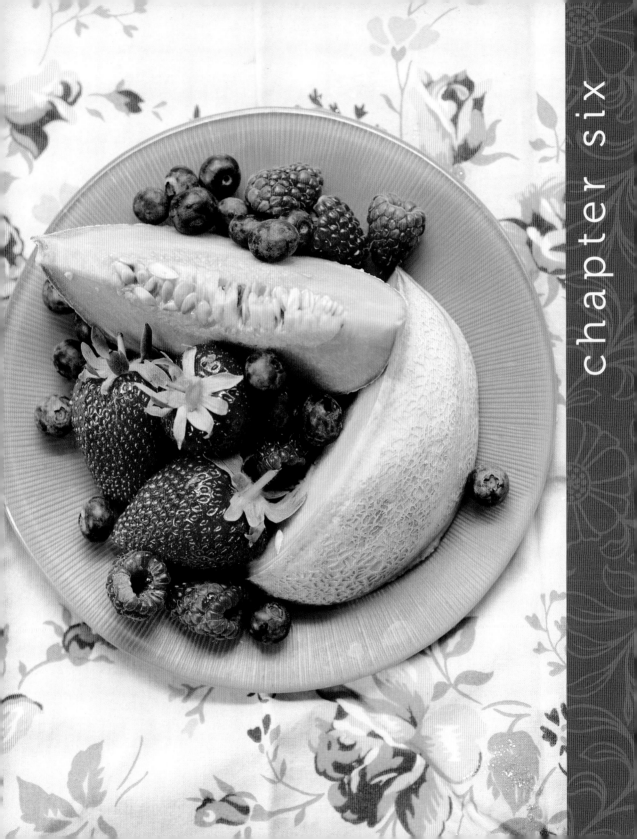

chapter six

Breakfasts

There's a reason why people say you should 'breakfast like a king' – without doubt, it's a crucial meal.

For years I skipped breakfast thinking that fewer calories first thing would result in me losing weight faster, and the chance to finally slide into a pair of size 10 jeans. I never felt particularly hungry when I woke up, and would pat myself on the back for resisting food first thing – only to be face down in the contents of a biscuit tin by 11am.

Eventually, it dawned on me that the reason I didn't feel hungry in the morning was because I'd stuffed myself the night before! And frankly, I was still pretty bloated.

Now, when I'm following **The Rules**, I eat lightly at night and wake up feeling better in the morning and ready for breakfast. If I'm off out and about, I'll grab a quick bowl of muesli or some porridge with a banana. If I've got more time on my hands then I'll go for some scrambled eggs with some smoked salmon. As long as you stick to **The Rules**, there are loads of filling breakfasts you can have and enjoy.

HERE ARE JUST A FEW TO GET YOU STARTED...

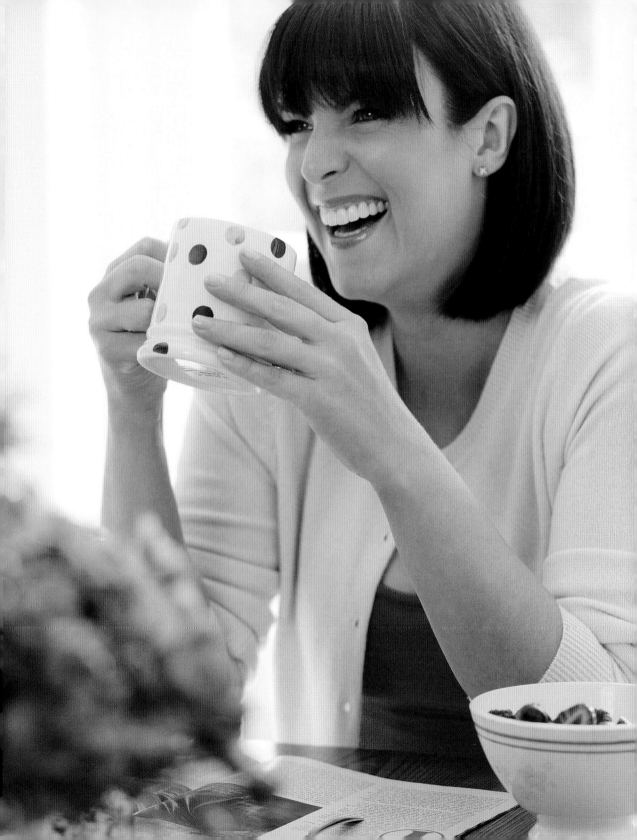

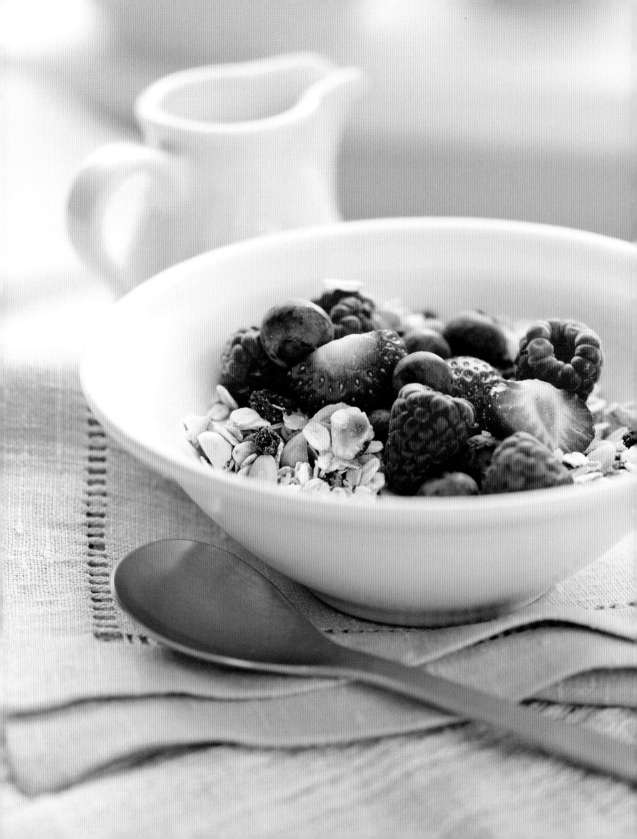

Summer Cereal

This combination makes a quick homemade breakfast cereal that you can knock together in minutes. Puffed rice can be found in most health-food stores – make sure it's sugar free. The dried fruit adds natural sweetness and the nuts give the cereal a good crunch. Eat this with milk from your daily allowance.

100g unsweetened puffed rice

100g jumbo oats

75g mixed dried fruit

25g flaked almonds

Makes 6 servings   Ready in under 5 minutes

1. Mix all the ingredients until thoroughly combined. Spoon a serving into a cereal bowl and pour over milk from your allowance. Store the rest in an airtight container for up to two weeks.

Homemade Muesli with Berries

Shop-bought muesli often contains sugar and sometimes includes a few cheeky wheat flakes too, so it's worth making your own. Kept in an airtight jar it will store for ages.

160g jumbo porridge oats

a handful (35g) mixed dried fruit

a handful (25g) roughly chopped mixed nuts

handful fresh berries, such as blueberries, raspberries and strawberries, or a mixture, to serve

Makes 5 servings   Ready in under 5 minutes

1. Toss the oats with the dried fruit and nuts in a lidded container.

2. Scoop 3–4 dessertspoons of the mixture into a bowl, top with berries and serve with milk from your 300ml daily allowance.

Fruity Porridge

You don't have to be Scottish to like porridge. I love it and I'm from Stoke-on-Trent. It makes a great breakfast – mainly because it'll stop you feeling hungry for hours.

4 heaped tbsp porridge oats (30g)

150ml semi-skimmed or skimmed milk, from your allowance

75ml cold water

1 medium banana

small handful mixed dried fruit (15g)

Serves 1   Ready in under 5 minutes

1. Put the porridge oats, milk and water in a small non-stick pan over a medium heat. Cook for 3–5 minutes or until the oats are tender and creamy, stirring frequently with a wooden spoon.

2. Pour into a bowl and top with sliced banana and mixed dried fruit. Add a splash of cold milk if you like and serve.

Or you could give one of these TREATS a try...

- **Cinnamon Porridge with Raisins**
  Stir a good pinch of ground cinnamon and a small handful of raisins into the porridge instead of the banana and mixed fruit topping.

- **Berries and Nuts Porridge**
  Top the porridge with a handful of fresh berries and a few roughly chopped nuts.

- **Lemon and Blueberry Porridge**
  Stir the finely grated zest of half a small lemon into the porridge as it cooks. Top with a splash of milk and a handful of fresh blueberries.

- **Apricot and Almond Porridge**
  Cut 3–4 no-soak apricots in half and put in a saucepan. Just cover with orange juice and cook gently for about 5 minutes until they are soft. Spoon apricots and juice over the porridge. Sprinkle with a few flaked almonds and serve.

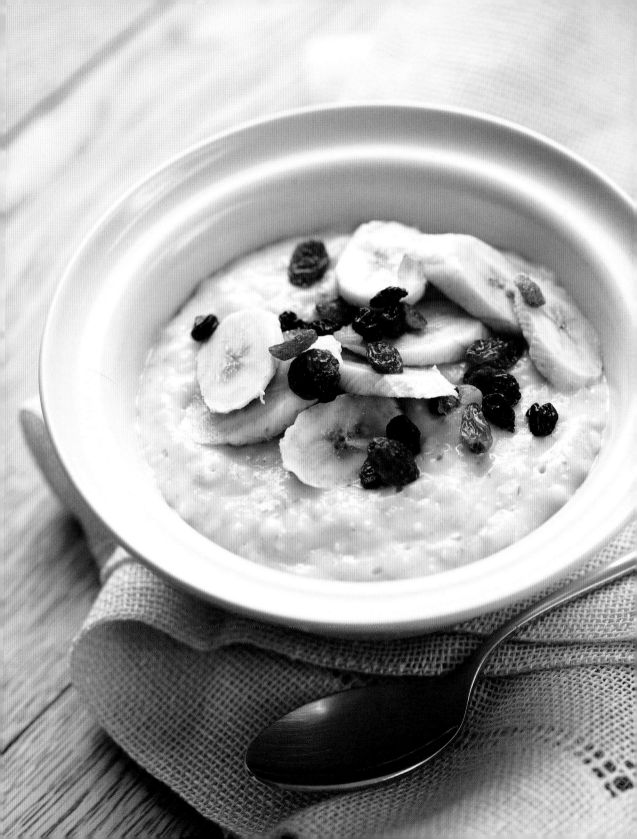

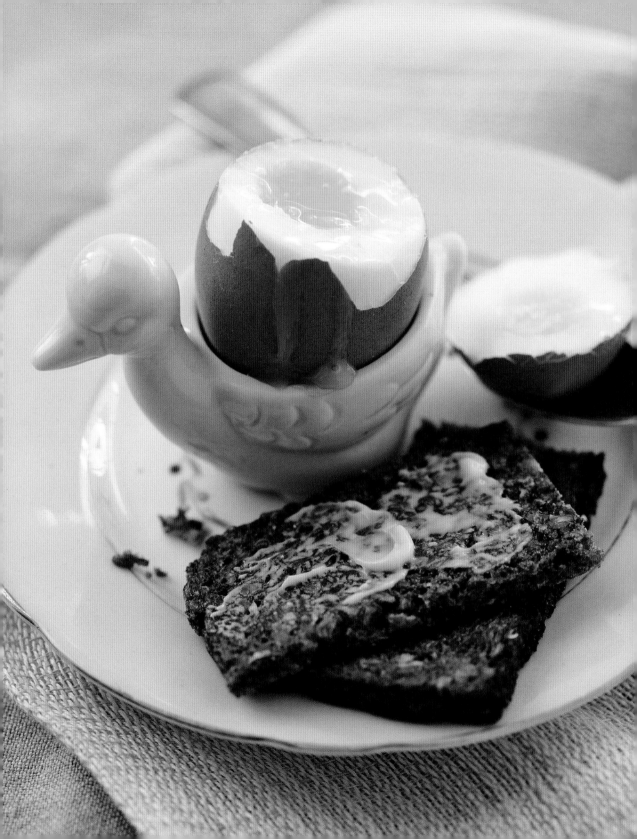

Boiled Egg and Soldiers

Come on, who doesn't love a boiled egg now and again?! Toasted rye bread, spread with a touch of sunflower or olive oil spread, is a good match for the egg and the whole thing is ready in less than 10 minutes. Only use the freshest free-range eggs.

If I'm using an egg straight from the fridge – and they should be stored in the fridge – I usually pop it into my bra to take the chill off while the water is coming to the boil. It will help prevent the shell cracking when it drops into the pan. Slightly weird I know, but it does seem to work – just make sure you don't hug anyone too closely while it's there.

I'm sure I don't need to tell you how to boil an egg, but mine always turn out pretty well anyway, so here's how I do it.

**1 large fresh
free-range egg**

**1 slice toasted rye
bread, spread lightly
with sunflower or olive
oil spread and cut
into fingers**

Serves 1   Ready in under 10 minutes

1. Half fill a small pan with water and bring to the boil.

2. Using a large spoon, gently drop the egg into the hot water and return to the boil. Boil for 6 minutes for a softly boiled egg, longer if you prefer something firmer. (Don't let the egg clunk about too much in the pan as it may crack the shell.)

3. Remove from the water with a slotted spoon, pop into an egg cup and serve with lightly toasted rye bread.

Scrambled Egg with Smoked Salmon and Watercress

I often have a small pack of smoked salmon in my fridge. It's perfect for quick breakfasts and lunches.

mild cooking oil spray

2 large free-range eggs, beaten

2 slices smoked salmon (40g), preferably wild or organic

small handful of watercress

Serves 1   Ready in under 5 minutes

1. Lightly mist a small saucepan with the oil and cook the eggs over a low heat for about a minute, stirring slowly with a wooden spoon, until creamy and only just set.

2. Fold the salmon onto a serving plate, add the watercress and spoon over the eggs. Season with a little freshly ground black pepper and serve.

Scrambled Egg on Rye Bread with Grilled Tomatoes

1 large ripe tomato, halved

mild cooking oil spray

1 large free-range egg, beaten

1 slice of rye bread spread very thinly with sunflower spread

Serves 1   Ready in under 10 minutes

1. Put the tomato halves on a grill pan, cut side up. Season with a little ground black pepper and cook under a preheated hot grill for 8–10 minutes until softened, checking occasionally.

2. Lightly mist a small saucepan with oil and cook the egg over a low heat for about a minute, stirring slowly with a wooden spoon, until creamy and only just set. Serve with rye bread.

Scrambled Eggs and Bacon

mild cooking oil spray

1 rasher rindless back
bacon (smoked or
unsmoked)

2 large free-range eggs,
beaten

1 rye crispbread
(optional)

Serves 1   Ready in under 5 minutes

1. Mist a small non-stick saucepan with oil and place over a
medium heat. Cut the bacon into strips and add to the pan. Cook
for about 2 minutes or until beginning to crisp. Reduce the heat.

2. Season the eggs with a little ground black pepper. Tip into the
pan with the bacon and cook for roughly 2 minutes, stirring very
slowly until they are cooked to your taste. Cooking the eggs over
a low heat will prevent them becoming stringy.

3. Put the crispbread on a plate and spoon the eggs and bacon
on top. Season with more pepper if liked and serve.

Mushrooms on Toast

I love mushrooms on toast and can't resist adding a squirt of tomato ketchup.
Add a rasher or two of fried or grilled bacon to this breakfast if you like.

small knob vegetable
spread

1tbsp sunflower oil

2 portobello mush-
rooms or a couple of
handfuls of closed cup
mushrooms, wiped and
thickly sliced

1 slice rye bread

Serves 1   Ready in under 5 minutes

1. Melt the vegetable spread with the oil in a non-stick frying pan
set over a high heat. Add the mushrooms and cook for 2–3
minutes until softened and lightly browned, stirring regularly.

2. Toast the rye bread and transfer to a plate. Season the
mushrooms with plenty of ground black pepper and tip over the
toast to serve.

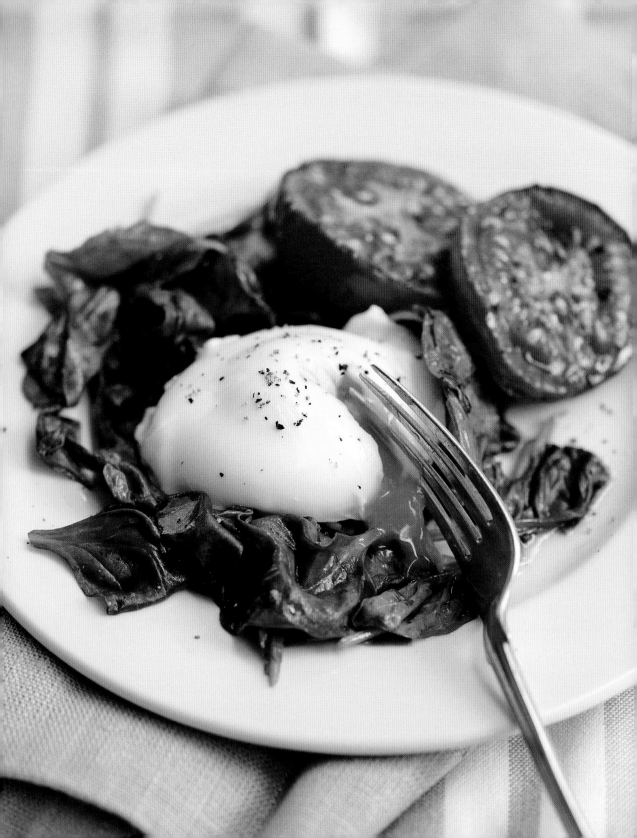

Poached Egg with Wilted Spinach and Grilled Tomato

I love a poached egg and this dish is particularly good for a late breakfast because it's served with grilled tomatoes and wilted spinach and feels a bit like a posh brunch. Serve with a mug of hot coffee for the full bistro vibe!

1 large ripe tomato, halved

1 large very fresh free-range egg

mild cooking oil spray

2 good handfuls baby spinach leaves

glass fresh orange or grapefruit juice, or 1 slice rye bread spread very thinly with sunflower spread, to serve

Serves 1   Ready in under 15 minutes

1. Put the tomato halves on a grill pan, cut side up. Season with a little ground black pepper and cook under a preheated hot grill for 8–10 minutes until softened, checking occasionally.

2. While the tomatoes are cooking, half fill a small pan with water and bring to the boil. Crack the egg into the water (or into a cup first if you prefer) and reduce the heat rapidly so that the water is only just bubbling. Cook for 3 minutes. If you have an egg poacher handy, forget the saucepan and use it!

3. Meanwhile, mist a small non-stick frying pan with the oil. Shake the spinach leaves into the pan and cook over a medium heat for 1–2 minutes or until just wilted, stirring frequently. Drain off any excess water and spoon the spinach into the centre of a plate.

4. Lift the egg from the pan using a slotted spoon and place on top of the spinach. Pop the grilled tomatoes beside it. Season with a little ground black pepper and serve with a glass of fresh orange or grapefruit juice or a slice of rye bread with sunflower or olive oil spread.

Pan-Fried Bacon with Mushrooms and Tomatoes

This is the perfect weekend breakfast – just double up the ingredients if you're making it for two. Settle down at the kitchen table with the papers, a hot cup of tea or coffee and enjoy.

mild cooking oil spray

2 rashers rindless lean back bacon, preferably dry-cured

small handful (6–8) small chestnut or button mushrooms, wiped and halved

5–6 cherry tomatoes, halved

good handful watercress or baby leaves

drizzle good quality balsamic vinegar

Serves 1   Ready in under 10 minutes

1. Mist a large non-stick frying pan with the oil and fry the bacon over a medium heat for 2–3 minutes until lightly browned.

2. Flip the bacon over and add the mushrooms to the pan. Mist with a little more cooking oil and continue frying together for a further 2–3 minutes, turning the mushrooms regularly until softened and golden around the edges.

3. Add the tomatoes to the pan and season with plenty of freshly ground black pepper. Cook with the bacon and mushrooms for about a minute until just beginning to soften, turning once.

4. Using a fork, take the bacon from the pan and arrange on a serving plate with the leaves. Scatter over the mushrooms and tomatoes. Drizzle with a dash of balsamic vinegar, season with a little more pepper and serve.

Anna's Tip

Transform this breakfast into a quick lunch by adding a freshly poached egg.

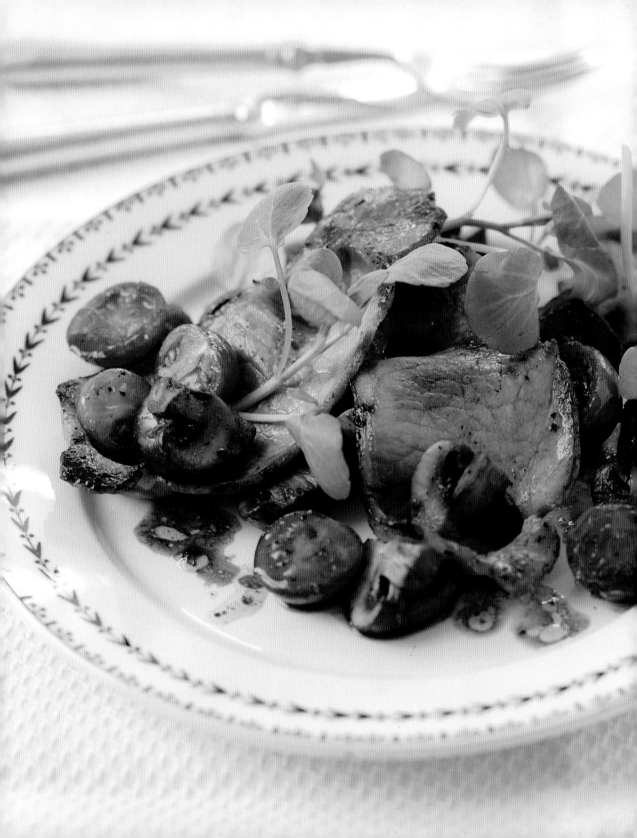

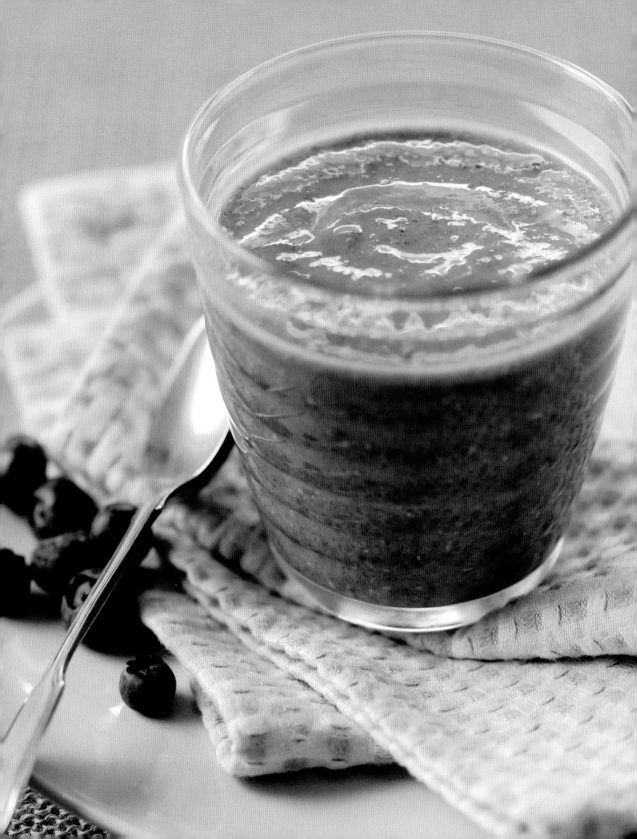

Berry Smoothie with Oats

Sometimes, all I crave for breakfast is something simple with fruit – especially when the weather's good. Because fruit is naturally sweet, I feel I've had a treat.

handful fresh
strawberries (100g),
hulled and halved

handful fresh raspberries
(50g)

1 small ripe banana,
thickly sliced

2 heaped tbsp porridge
oats (15g)

splash semi-skimmed
or skimmed milk from
your allowance

Serves 1   Ready in under 5 minutes

1. Put the berries, banana and oats in a blender, food processor or smoothie maker. Add the milk and blend until as smooth as possible. Add a little extra milk if it still seems too thick.

2. Pour into a tall glass, using a spatula to scrape every last bit out of the blender. Drink or use a spoon to serve.

Zesty Fruit Salad

A really good fruit salad is my idea of heaven and makes a great breakfast or snack, anytime. Feel free to chuck in any fruit you fancy.

1 small ripe pineapple

1 large ripe mango

2 large kiwi fruit

2 apples

2 oranges

1 lime

Serves 6   Ready in under 10 minutes

1. Peel the pineapple and cut into quarters lengthways. Cut out the central core and discard. Cut the pineapple into pieces and put in a bowl. Peel the mango and cut in half either side of the large, flat stone. Slice the mango and add to the pineapple.

2. Peel and slice the kiwi fruit. Quarter, core and slice the apples. Peel and segment the oranges. Add to the rest of the fruit. Finely grate the lime and squeeze the juice. Stir into the fruit and serve.

Lunches

Like any sane person with an appetite I love a long lunch. Sometimes there just isn't enough time, particularly if you work in an office. But with a little bit of organisation and a well-stocked fridge I know that there are tons of foods for me to enjoy. So now I can choose to either cook a simple hot meal or make something that can be easily packed up, whacked in a plastic pot and eaten on the go.

I discovered open-topped sandwiches a while ago and they've totally changed the way I look at the traditional 'sarnie'. For years, I'd been ramming fillings between two thick slices of flabby white bread, or buying massive baguettes saturated with butter. I nearly cried with joy when paninis became popular in all the coffee shops and every lunchtime I'd scoff the largest, cheesiest one on offer without even thinking. Is it any wonder I got fat?

Carbs are a comfort food for me and it's brilliant to know that these recipes can be knocked up really easily – I can eat creamy risotto and spicy noodles and still lose weight. Give these ideas a go and see for yourself.

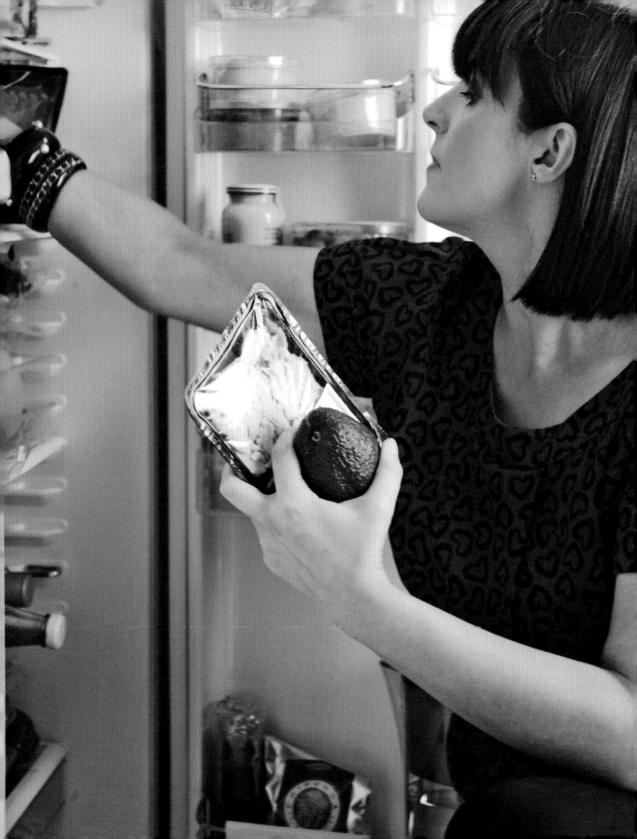

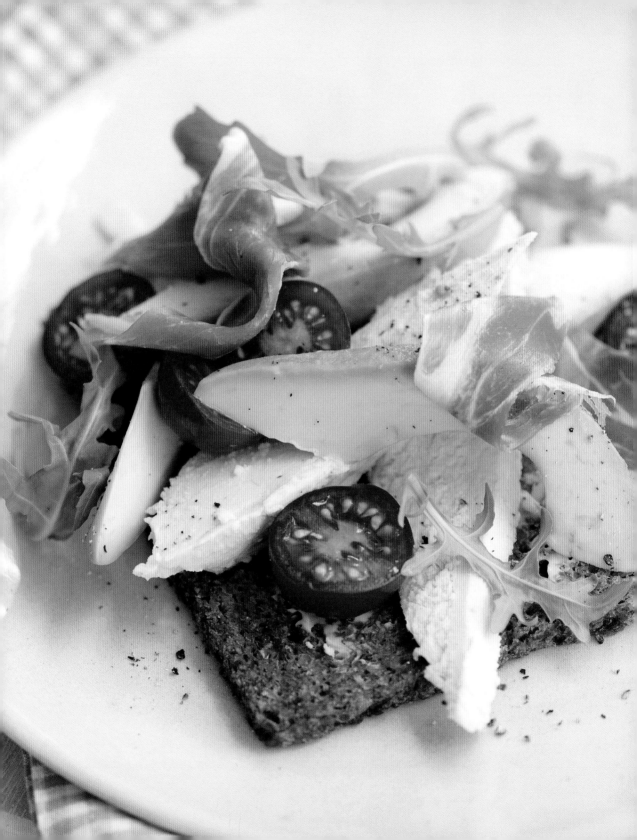

Roast Chicken with Parma Ham and Avocado

One of my favourite lunches and oh, so simple. Put all the bits in a lunch box and you can even assemble it at work if you want to.

1 slice rye bread

½tsp sunflower
or olive oil spread

½ small ripe avocado

½ skinless roast chicken
breast (50g)

handful cherry tomatoes

1 slice Parma ham

handful rocket leaves

lemon wedge, to serve

Serves 1   Ready in under 5 minutes

1. Spread the rye bread very thinly with sunflower or olive oil spread and put on a plate. Stone the avocado and cut into thin slices. Strip off and discard the skin. Slice the chicken and cut the tomatoes in half.

2. Place the avocado, chicken, tomatoes and Parma ham on the rye bread with a few rocket leaves. Squeeze over a little fresh lemon juice and season with plenty of freshly ground black pepper.

Or you could try one of these IDEAS instead...

- **Ham and Egg with Cress**
  Spread 1 slice of rye bread very thinly with sunflower or olive oil spread and top with 1 hard-boiled egg, sliced, 2 slices ham and 1 tomato, quartered. Drizzle with 2tsp salad cream and sprinkle with a handful of freshly snipped cress. **Serves 1.**

- **Roast Beef and Watercress**
  Spread 1 slice of rye bread very thinly with sunflower or olive oil spread and 1tsp hot horseradish sauce. Top with 2 slices rare roast beef, 3 cherry tomatoes, halved, and a few sprigs fresh watercress. **Serves 1.**

Smoked Salmon with Watercress and Lemon

Smoked salmon goes brilliantly with rye bread. Try gravadlax or even some flaked smoked trout when you fancy a change.

1 slice rye bread

½tsp sunflower or olive oil spread

4 slices smoked salmon (about 90g)

large handful watercress

lemon wedge, to serve

Serves 1   Ready in under 5 minutes

1. Spread the rye bread very thinly with sunflower or olive oil spread and cut in half.

2. Put the rye bread on a plate and top with the smoked salmon and watercress. Season with freshly ground black pepper. Serve the salmon with a lemon wedge for squeezing over.

Or you could try one of these IDEAS instead...

- **Prawn and Avocado**

  Mix a handful (50g) cooked, peeled prawns (thawed) with 1tbsp salad cream and ½tsp tomato ketchup. Arrange ½ sliced avocado and a handful baby gem lettuce leaves on a plate and spoon the prawns over. Serve with a slice of rye bread and a wedge of lemon for squeezing over. **Serves 1.**

- **Tuna with Tomatoes and Salad Cream**

  Put 3 rye crispbreads on a plate with 3–4 crunchy lettuce leaves or a handful of rocket. Top with 1 x 80g can tuna in oil or water, drained and flaked into chunky pieces. Add a handful of cherry tomatoes, halved, and drizzle with 2–3tsp salad cream. **Serves 1.**

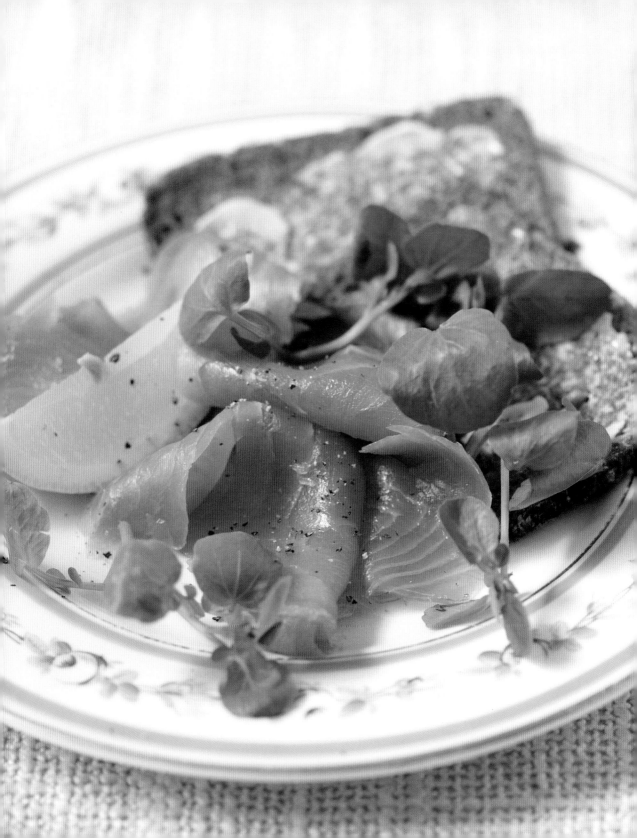

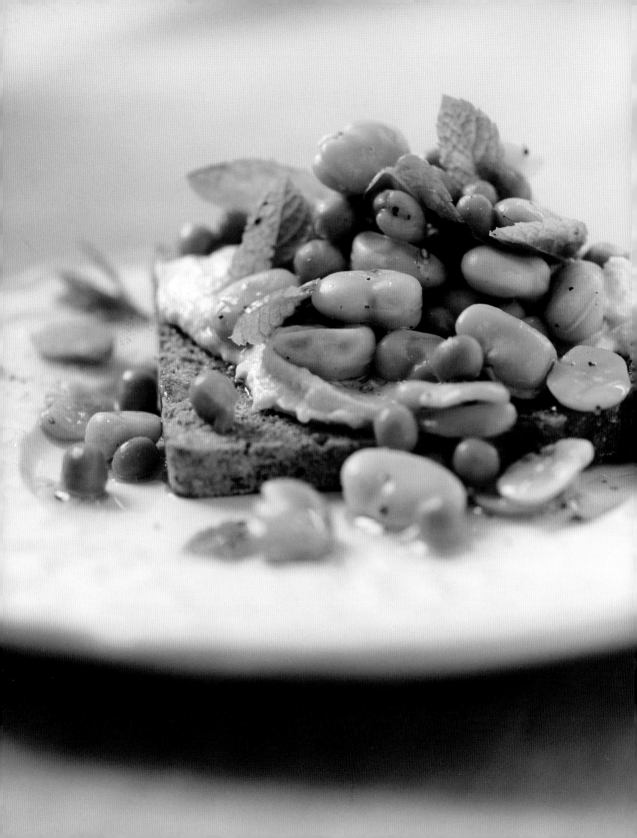

Houmous and Minted Beans

OK, so this one takes a little more time. But the combination of creamy houmous and minted beans is definitely worth five more minutes.

2 handfuls (100g) frozen broad beans

2 handfuls (50g) frozen peas

handful small fresh mint leaves

2tsp extra virgin olive oil

1tsp freshly squeezed lemon juice

2 slices rye bread

4tbsp reduced-fat houmous

Serves 2   Ready in under 10 minutes

1. Half fill a small pan with water and bring to the boil. Add the beans and peas and return to the boil. Cook for 2 minutes.

2. Drain the vegetables in a sieve and rinse under running water until cold. Slip the skins off half the beans by opening each one gently and popping the bean out. Discard the skins and put all the beans and peas in a small bowl.

3. Add the mint leaves to the vegetables and pour over the oil and lemon juice. Season with a little salt and plenty of freshly ground black pepper.

4. Spread 2 pieces of rye bread thickly with the houmous. Put on 2 plates and pile the minted vegetables and their dressing on top. Serve immediately.

Or you could try one of these IDEAS instead...

- **Roasted Peppers and Houmous**
  Spread 3 rye crispbreads or 1 slice rye bread with 3tbsp reduced-fat houmous and top with a handful of rocket leaves and 75g chargrilled peppers, drained. **Serves 1.**

- **Avocado, Rocket and Tomato**
  Put 3 rye crispbreads or 1 slice rye bread on a plate and top with a handful of rocket, a few cherry tomatoes, halved, a handful of marinated olives and ½ avocado, sliced. Drizzle with a little balsamic vinegar. **Serves 1.**

Chicken Laksa

This isn't a really authentic laksa, but it's got a delicious creamy coconut sauce, fragrant flavours and yummy rice noodles. Diet. What diet?

mild cooking oil spray

2tbsp finely chopped ginger (about a thumb of fresh root ginger)

2 garlic cloves, peeled and finely chopped

400ml can of reduced-fat coconut milk

½ chicken stock cube

1 red chilli, deseeded and cut into tiny pieces

2 skinless, boneless free-range chicken breasts, cut into thin strips

1 pack (about 300g) stir-fry vegetables

2 bundles (120g) dry rice noodles, preferably the wide ones

3–4 Kaffir lime leaves (optional)

fresh coriander or basil leaves (optional)

Serves 4 Ready in under 15 minutes

1. Mist a large non-stick saucepan with cooking oil and gently fry the ginger and garlic for 2–3 minutes, stirring constantly.

2. Pour the coconut milk into the pan and then refill the can with cold water twice, stirring into the coconut milk each time.

3. Crumble over the stock cube and stir in the chilli. Bring to a simmer and cook for a couple of minutes before adding the chicken, vegetables and noodles. Add 3–4 Kaffir lime leaves if you have some.

4. Return to a simmer and cook for a further 4–5 minutes or until the chicken is cooked, stirring occasionally. Season to taste with salt and pepper. (If you have any fresh coriander or basil leaves handy, scatter a few over now.) Stand for 4–5 minutes.

5. Ladle into deep bowls and devour.

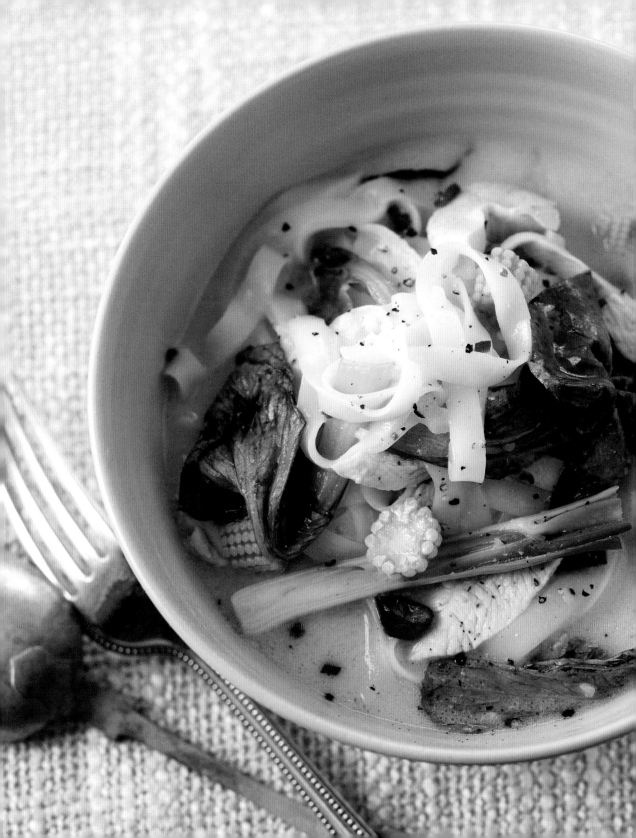

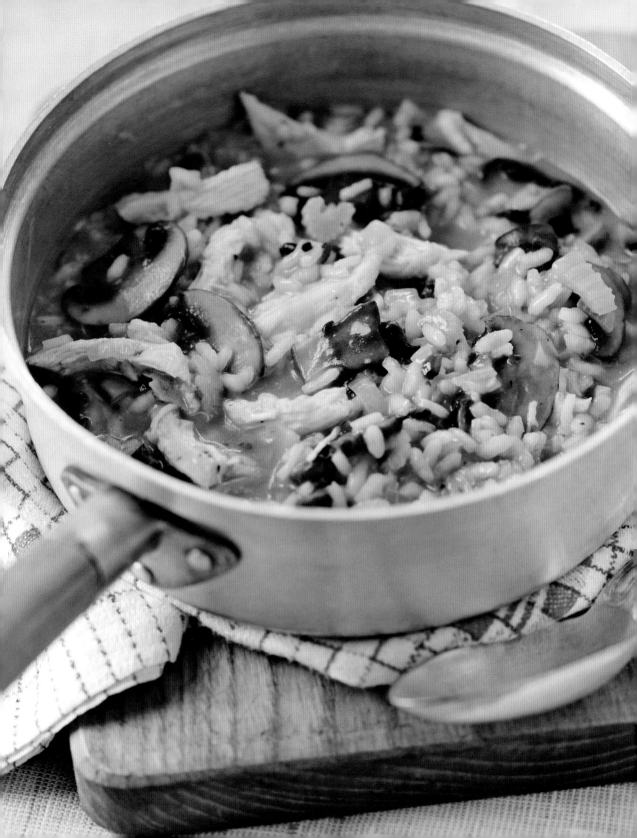

Easy Chicken and Mushroom Risotto

The perfect lunch on a cold day, this is probably the easiest chicken risotto you'll ever make. There's none of that adding the stock ladle by ladle – I just pour it all in at the same time, and it still works brilliantly. As long as you stir it regularly, the rice should be creamy and tender.

2tsp olive oil

1 medium onion, peeled and finely chopped

1 garlic clove, peeled and finely chopped

1 stick celery, trimmed and thinly sliced

75g (10–12) chestnut mushrooms, wiped and sliced

75g (roughly ¼ mug) Arborio risotto rice

450ml hot chicken stock (fresh or made with a cube)

1 skinless, boneless, cooked chicken breast, torn into pieces

Serves 2   Ready in under 30 minutes

1. Heat the oil in a medium non-stick saucepan and gently fry the onion, garlic and celery for 6–8 minutes until softened, stirring occasionally.

2. Add the mushrooms and fry with the vegetables for a further 3 minutes, stirring. Tip the rice into the pan and stir for a few seconds.

3. Carefully pour over the stock, stir well and bring to a simmer. Cook for 15–18 minutes, stirring regularly until the rice is almost tender and the sauce is creamy.

4. Add the chicken pieces and heat through in the hot rice for 3 minutes, stirring constantly. (If the risotto looks a little dry at any stage, simply add a touch more stock.) Spoon into warmed bowls to serve.

Anna's Tip

For a veggie version, simply make the risotto with vegetable stock, leave out the chicken and add a handful of frozen peas or broad beans.

Char-grilled Pepper and Bean Tortilla

You'll need a small non-stick, flame-proof frying pan for this recipe. This tortilla can be served warm with salad for lunch or supper, or cooled and wrapped in greaseproof paper for a mouth-watering packed lunch. Using beans instead of potatoes gives it a great texture and makes this tortilla extra delicious. When your two weeks are up, feel free to add a few cubes of feta or goat's cheese to the mix.

mild cooking oil spray

½ medium onion, peeled and finely diced

1 garlic clove, peeled and crushed

280g jar char-grilled peppers in oil, drained well and cut into chunks

400g can butterbeans or cannellini beans, drained and rinsed

good handful frozen peas

5 large free-range eggs

good pinch dried mixed herbs

Serves 4   Ready in under 15 minutes

1. Mist a small non-stick, flameproof frying pan with oil and gently fry the onion for 4–5 minutes until softened, stirring occasionally. Add the garlic, pepper pieces, beans and peas and fry for a further 2 minutes, stirring.

2. Whisk the eggs and mixed herbs in a bowl and season with a little salt and freshly ground black pepper.

3. Pour the egg mixture over the fried vegetables and stir a couple of times. Cook over a low heat for a further 3–4 minutes without stirring until the egg is almost set. Meanwhile, preheat the grill to hot.

4. Place the frying pan under the grill and cook for a further 2–3 minutes or until the egg mixture is set and lightly browned. Remove from the heat and leave to cool for 2–3 minutes before turning out onto a chopping board. Cut into thick wedges to serve.

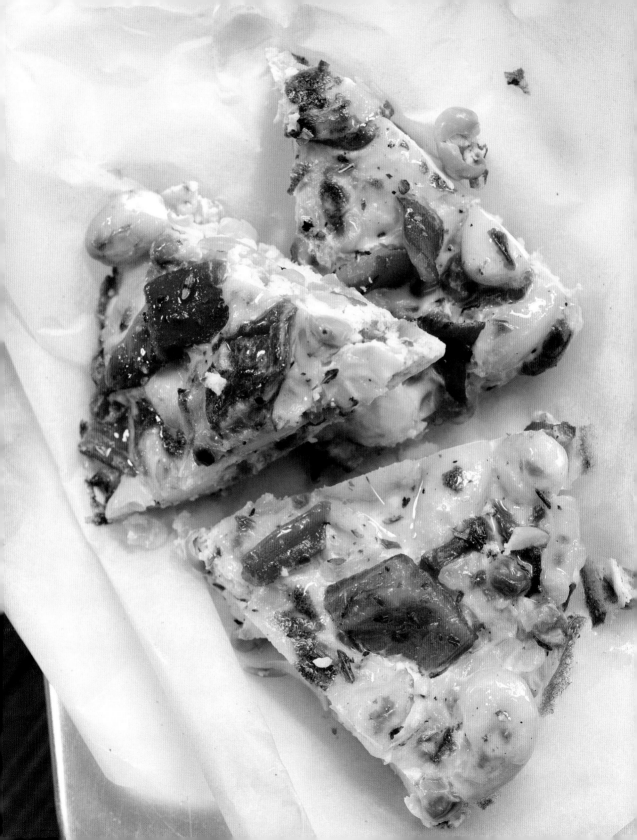

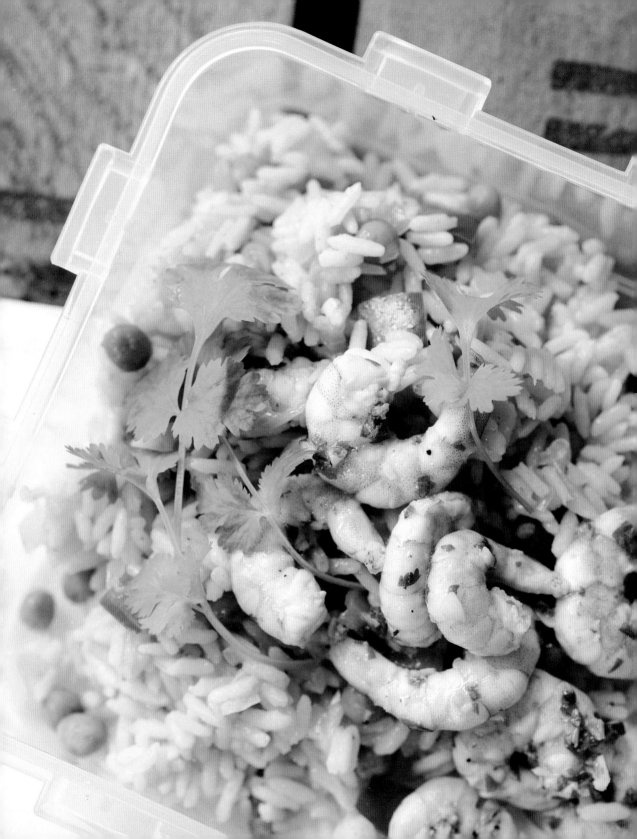

Spiced Rice and Garlic Prawns

This rice salad is great just as it is, but tastes even better when combined with the marinated prawns. Make sure you cool the cooked rice quickly and then keep it cold before serving.

1 tbsp sunflower oil

1 small onion, peeled and finely chopped

1 red pepper, deseeded and diced

1 garlic clove, peeled and crushed

75g easy-cook long grain rice

1–2tsp mild curry powder

½tsp ground turmeric

600ml water

½ chicken or vegetable stock cube

50g frozen peas

FOR THE PRAWNS

200g large cooked peeled prawns, thawed if frozen

½ small garlic clove, peeled and crushed

1tbsp chopped fresh parsley or coriander leaves

freshly squeezed lemon juice, to taste

Serves 2   Ready in under 45 minutes

1. For the rice, heat the oil in a medium non-stick saucepan and gently fry the onion and pepper for 5 minutes or until softened and lightly coloured, stirring regularly.

2. Add the garlic and rice and cook for a few seconds before stirring in the curry powder and turmeric. Pour in the water, crumble over the stock cube and bring to the boil.

3. Cook the rice for 10 minutes or until tender, stirring occasionally and adding the peas for the last 2 minutes of cooking time. Drain the rice and vegetables in a colander then spread over a large plate to cool quickly. When the rice is cool, fluff up the grains and transfer to a serving dish or two lidded containers if you are planning a packed lunch.

4. Put the prawns in a bowl and add a little garlic, the parsley or coriander and a squeeze of lemon juice. Season with freshly ground black pepper and toss well together. Spoon on top of the rice. Cover and keep cold in the fridge. Pack with ice blocks if eating on the move.

Chilli con Carne

I love a good chilli and often cook it with vegetarian Quorn mince, which I reckon is just as good as the real thing.

300g lean minced beef

1 medium onion, peeled and finely chopped

2 garlic cloves, peeled and finely chopped

1–2tsp hot chilli powder

½tsp ground cumin

½tsp dried mixed herbs

400g can chopped tomatoes

2tbsp tomato puree

1 beef stock cube

400g can red kidney beans, rinsed and drained

1tbsp cornflour

6 palmfuls easy-cook long grain rice (210g)

fresh coriander, to serve

Serves 6   Ready in under 1 hour

1. Fry the mince with the onion and garlic in a large non-stick saucepan over a medium heat for about 5 minutes or until the beef is no longer pink – there's no need to use any additional oil. Stir the meat with a wooden spoon to break up any large clumps. Sprinkle over the spices and herbs and cook for a minute or so more, stirring continuously.

2. Add the tomatoes and tomato puree. Refill the tomato can with cold water and pour into the pan. Crumble the stock cube over the top, season with salt and a few twists of ground black pepper, give a good stir and bring to a simmer.

3. When the liquid is bubbling, but not too madly, cover the pan loosely with a lid and leave to simmer over a low heat for 20 minutes, stirring occasionally. Stir in the beans, cover loosely and cook for a further 15–20 minutes or until the beef is tender.

4. Mix the cornflour with a tablespoon of cold water in a small bowl and stir into the chilli. Continue simmering without a lid for a further 3–4 minutes until the sauce is thick, stirring regularly. Serve with freshly boiled rice if eating for lunch. Sprinkle with a little freshly chopped coriander if you have some.

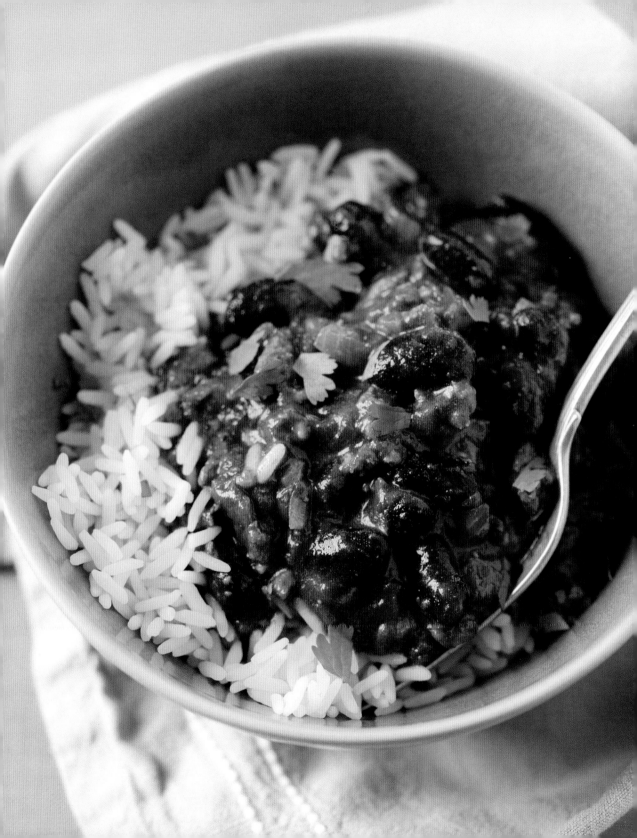

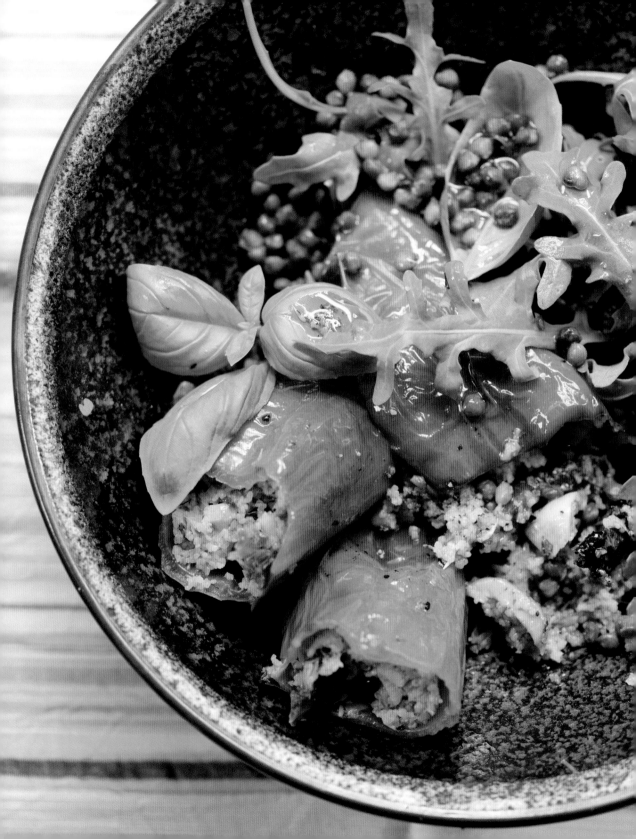

Couscous and Vegetable Stuffed Peppers

These peppers are a cinch to make and taste amazing. They also reheat really well if they're not eaten at once. I like to serve mine with a dressed green salad tossed with a few cooked puy lentils. Choose squarish red peppers as they'll stand better when roasting.

50g barley couscous

4 red peppers or
2 Romano peppers
(the long ones)

8 pitted green olives,
quartered

2 spring onions,
trimmed and sliced

8 SunBlush (semi-dried)
tomato pieces in oil,
drained (reserving the oil)

4 char-grilled artichokes
in oil, drained and
roughly chopped

15g toasted flaked
almonds

15g sultanas

freshly squeezed juice
and finely grated zest
½ small lemon

small bunch roughly
chopped fresh mint
leaves

small bunch chopped
fresh coriander leaves

Serves 4   Ready in under 1 hour

1. Put the couscous in a bowl and pour over 50ml just-boiled water. Leave to stand for 5 minutes. Cut the top off each pepper and retain. Scrape out the seeds and any white membrane. Preheat the oven to 200°C/Gas 6.

2. Fluff up the couscous with a fork then stir in the olives, spring onions, tomato pieces, artichokes, almonds and sultanas. Add 1tbsp of the reserved tomato oil, lemon juice and zest, chopped mint and coriander leaves. Season with freshly ground black pepper and a little salt if necessary.

3. Stuff the mixture into the peppers ensuring it is packed fairly tightly. Place the lids back on top and put on a foil-lined baking tray. The red peppers will be able to stand upright but the Romano peppers will need to be placed on their sides.

4. Bake in the centre of the oven for 25–30 minutes or until the peppers are soft and the filling is hot. Serve with a large mixed salad.

Spinach and Tomato Omelette

It's easy to rustle up a quick omelette for a tasty lunch in less than ten minutes. And it's definitely worth forking out for a decent non-stick frying pan!

mild cooking oil spray

3 medium
free-range eggs

2 ripe tomatoes,
quartered

handful baby
spinach leaves

Serves 1   Ready in under 10 minutes

1. Mist a small non-stick frying pan with the oil and place over a medium heat. Break the eggs into a bowl and beat with a large metal whisk. Season with salt and pepper.

2. Pour the eggs into the frying pan. As the eggs begin to set, use a wooden spoon to draw the cooked egg towards the centre 4–5 times, working your way around the pan.

3. Scatter the tomatoes and spinach leaves over and leave to cook for a further 2–3 minutes until the eggs are just set, the tomatoes are warm and the spinach is beginning to wilt.

4. Season with more freshly ground black pepper and carefully fold the omelette over. Slide onto a warmed plate and serve.

Or you could give one of these FILLINGS a try instead...

- **Leek and Pea**
  Lightly fry a small leek, trimmed and sliced, until softened, adding a handful of frozen peas for the last couple of minutes cooking time. Pour the beaten eggs over and cook as above for about 5 minutes until just set.

- **Prawn and Chive**
  Stir 1tbsp of snipped chives into the egg and cook as above, adding a handful of thawed, cooked peeled prawns to the pan in Step 3.

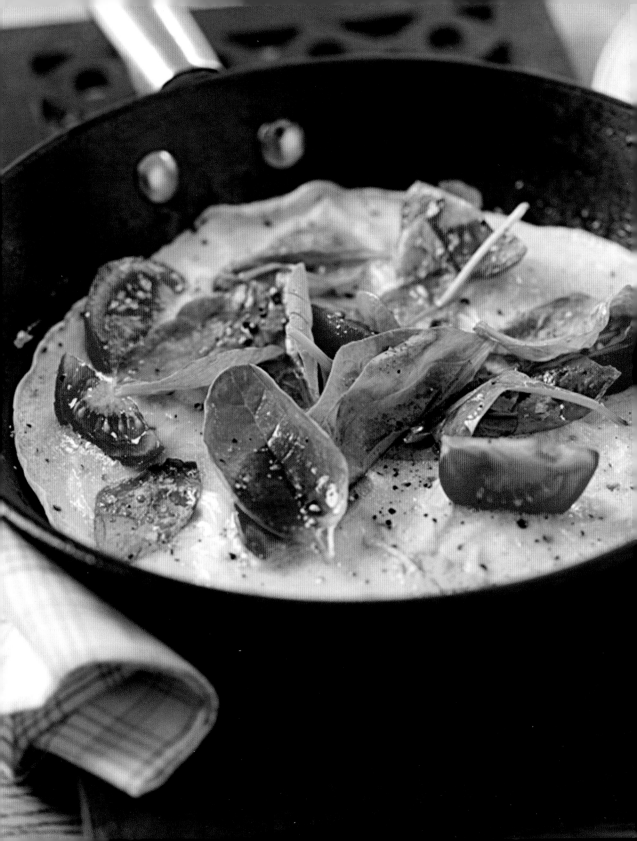

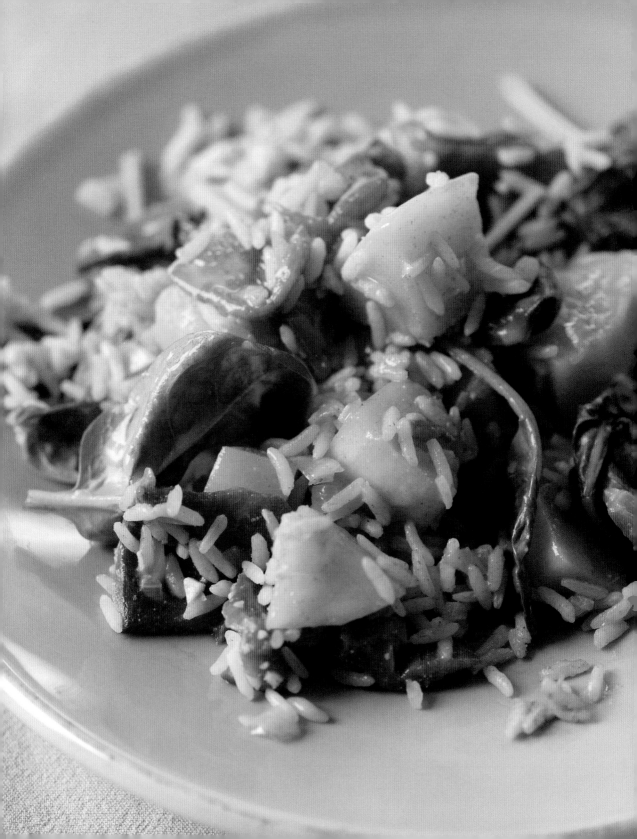

Moroccan Spiced Butternut Squash with Rice and Roasted Peppers

This is one of my favourites. I'm really into Moroccan flavours – they're the perfect way to spice up stews and soups. And this dish is all made in one pan. What's not to love?!

1tbsp sunflower oil

1 small onion, peeled and finely chopped

2 garlic cloves, peeled and finely chopped

½ medium butternut squash (roughly 450g)

1tsp each ground coriander, cumin and hot chilli powder

¼tsp ground cinnamon

good pinch saffron threads

125g (roughly ½ mug) easy cook long grain rice

700ml just-boiled water

290g jar char-grilled peppers in oil, drained

freshly squeezed juice ½ lemon

4 large handfuls baby spinach leaves, washed

Serves 4 **Ready in under 30 minutes**

1. Heat the sunflower oil in a large saucepan, or flameproof casserole, and gently fry the onion and garlic for 5 minutes, stirring occasionally. Peel and deseed the squash and cut into roughly 2cm chunks.

2. Sprinkle all the spices into the pan with the onion and cook for a few seconds before adding the squash and rice. Pour over the water, stir well and bring to a simmer. Cook for 12 minutes over a medium heat, stirring occasionally.

3. Cut the peppers into chunky pieces and add to the pan. Cook with the vegetables and rice for a further 3–4 minutes, or until the squash is softened, the rice is tender and most of the liquid has been absorbed. Stir regularly towards the end of the cooking time and add a little extra water if necessary.

4. Pour over the lemon juice and add the spinach leaves. Toss together over a low heat for 1–2 minutes until the spinach leaves wilt. Season to taste with salt and freshly ground black pepper. Serve with a large, lightly dressed salad.

Soups

I'm a bit obsessed with soup. I always keep soup stashed in the fridge or freezer because I know that it'll hit the spot for me when I need it most. If I'm feeling hungry after work, a quick bowl of soup always takes the edge off those pangs and stops me snacking on the wrong kind of food before dinner.

I sometimes have soup for lunch with a slice of rye bread and a simple salad, or just warm up a bowl for my evening meal if I'm not feeling particularly hungry. If you don't have the time to make your own soup, you can pick up fresh soup in cartons really easily and some are great. Make sure you stay well away from any containing ingredients that don't conform to **The Rules** though.

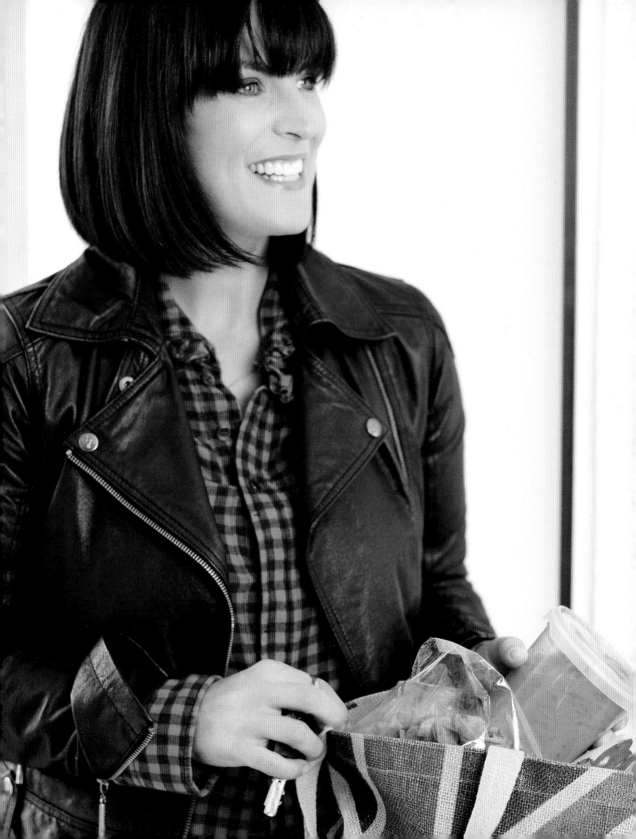

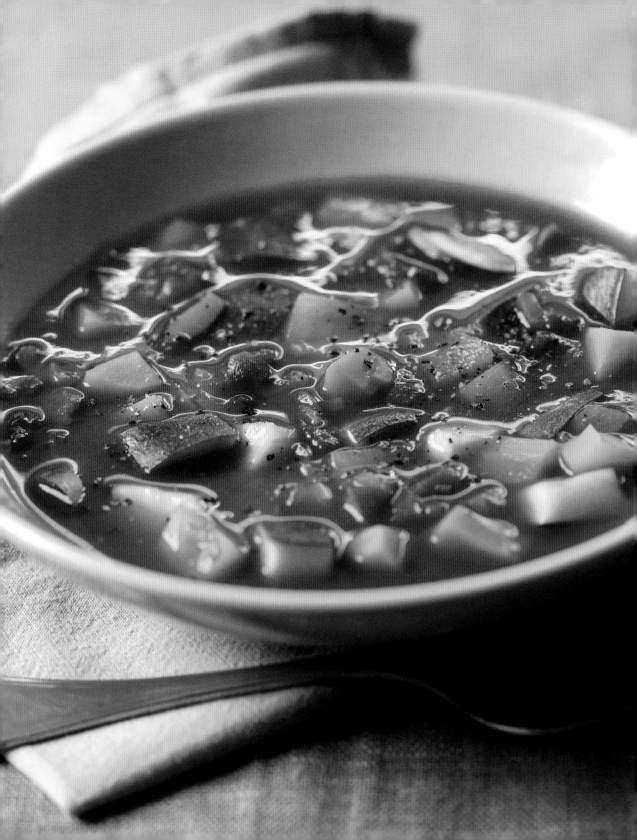

Chunky Vegetable Soup

I swear by this sort of soup for helping me lose weight. It's dead easy to chuck together, keeps well in the fridge and tastes great. The best thing about this soup is that you can eat it at any time whenever you're feeling a little bit peckish.

1 litre cold water

1 vegetable or chicken stock cube

400g can chopped tomatoes with herbs

1tbsp tomato puree

1 medium onion, peeled and finely chopped

2 garlic cloves, peeled and crushed

2 medium carrots, peeled and diced

1 red pepper, deseeded and diced

1 yellow pepper, deseeded and diced

2 medium courgettes, trimmed and diced

Makes 6 servings   Ready in under 25 minutes

1. Pour the water into a large saucepan and bring to a simmer. Crumble over the stock cube and stir until dissolved.

2. Add all the remaining ingredients, except the courgettes, and return to a simmer. The water should be bubbling at a fairly fast rate without boiling.

3. Simmer the vegetables for 5 minutes, then add the courgettes and continue simmering for a further 8–10 minutes or until all the vegetables are tender, stirring occasionally.

4. Season with lots of freshly ground black pepper.

Anna's Tip

If you prefer smooth soups, simply cool the contents of the pan, then transfer to a blender or food processor and blitz to a puree. Tip back into the saucepan and stir in extra water.

Carrot and Coriander Soup

I used to spend a fortune on cartons of carrot and coriander soup, but this one tastes loads better than the shop-bought versions and contains no hidden extras.

mild cooking oil spray

1 medium onion, peeled and finely chopped

2 garlic cloves, peeled and crushed

1 tsp ground coriander

6 medium carrots, peeled and coarsely grated

1.2 litres cold water

1 vegetable or chicken stock cube

1 small bunch (about 20g) fresh coriander

Makes 4 servings   Ready in under 25 minutes

1. Mist a large, deep saucepan with cooking oil spray. Gently fry the onion for 2–3 minutes, stirring. Add the garlic and sprinkle over the ground coriander. Cook together for 2 minutes more, stirring.

2. Tip the carrots into the pan, pour over the water and add the stock cube. Bring to the boil and cook for 10 minutes or until the carrots are very tender, stirring occasionally. Remove from the heat and blitz with a stick blender until smooth. (Watch out for splashes as the soup will be extremely hot.)

3. Finely chop the coriander leaves and stir into the soup just before serving. Season the soup to taste with salt and pepper. Ladle into deep bowls and serve.

Anna's Tip

Grating the carrots means they'll cook quicker, but you can always finely chop them if you prefer.

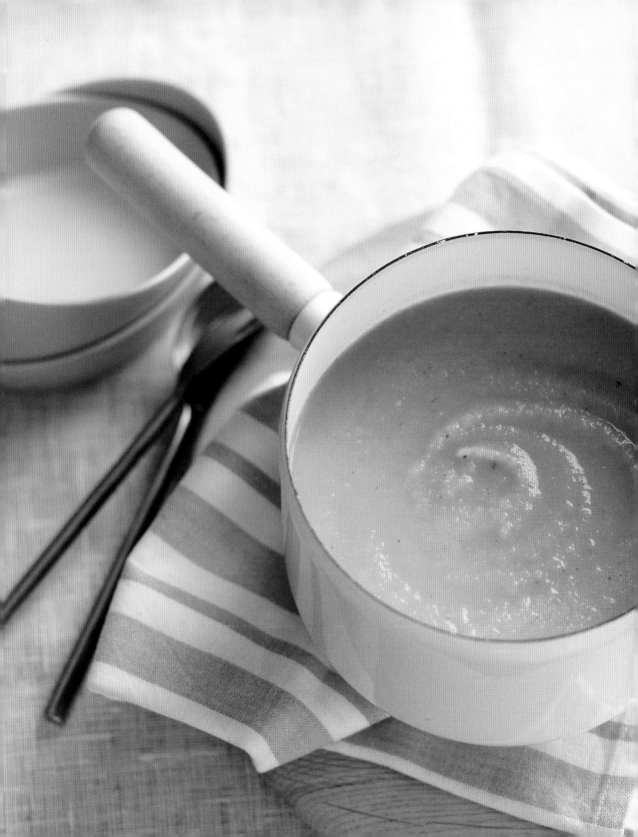

Curried Lentil Soup

Spicy food always makes me feel more satisfied and this combination of lightly curried lentils and vegetables is a great soup to bung in a flask and take to work.

1 medium onion, peeled

3 medium carrots, peeled

2 sticks celery, trimmed

2tsp sunflower oil

2tsp medium curry powder

150g (roughly ½ mug) dried red lentils, rinsed

1 litre cold water

1 vegetable or chicken stock cube

Makes 4 servings

Ready in under 30 minutes

1. Roughly chop the onion and carrots. Thinly slice the celery. Heat the oil in a large saucepan. Add the onion and curry powder to the pan and fry gently for 5 minutes or until the onion is softened, stirring regularly.

2. Tip the lentils into the pan and stir in the carrots, celery, water and stock cube. Bring to a simmer and cook for 15 minutes or until the lentils are completely softened, stirring regularly.

3. Remove the pan from the heat and use a stick blender to blitz until smooth. (Watch out for splashes as the soup will be extremely hot.) Add salt and pepper to taste. Return to the hob and warm through gently, stirring occasionally.

Creamy Mushroom Soup

This is the best homemade mushroom soup I have ever tasted. Use milk from your daily allowance to make it.

mild cooking oil spray

300g chestnut or closed cup mushrooms, wiped and sliced

1 medium onion, peeled and roughly chopped

1 garlic clove, peeled and crushed

600ml water

1 chicken or vegetable stock cube

200ml skimmed or semi-skimmed cow's milk

Makes 4 servings   Ready in under 30 minutes

1. Mist a large saucepan with cooking oil and fry the mushrooms over a high heat for 2–3 minutes until lightly browned, stirring frequently. Tip into a bowl and set aside.

2. Return the pan to a medium heat and mist with more cooking oil. Add the onion and cook for 5 minutes until softened, stirring regularly. Scatter over the garlic and cook with the onion for a further minute, stirring.

3. Add the mushrooms along with 600ml cold water and the stock cube. Bring to the boil, stirring to dissolve the stock cube, then reduce the heat slightly and simmer for 10 minutes.

4. Remove the pan from the heat and allow to cool for 5 minutes. Use a stick blender to blitz until smooth. (Watch out for splashes as the soup will be extremely hot.) Slowly stir in the milk, return to the hob and warm through gently without boiling, stirring regularly. Season with freshly ground black pepper.

Anna's Tip

If you don't have a stick blender, cool the soups then blitz in a blender or food processor until smooth. Return to the pan and warm through gently before serving.

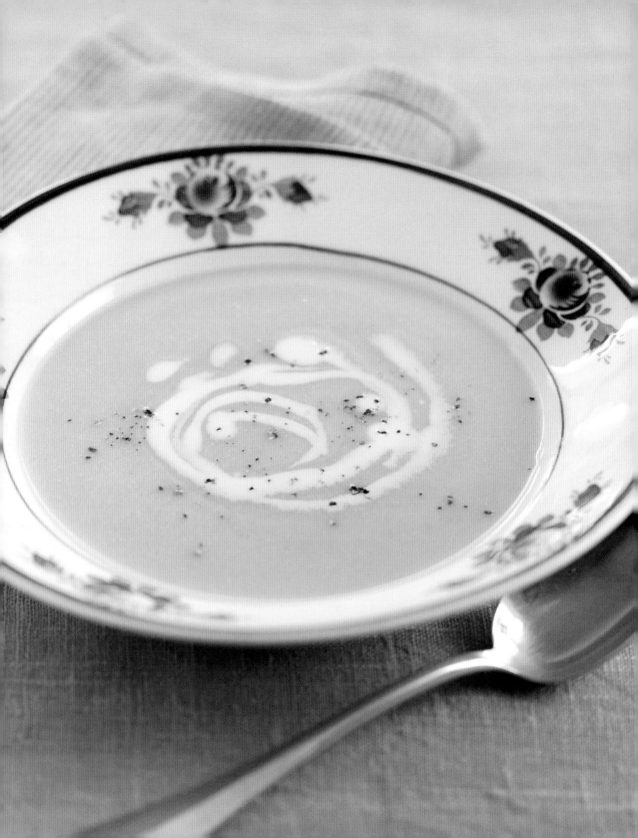

Butternut Squash and Coconut Soup

I LOVE this soup. And whenever I make it my friends think I actually know something about cooking! Save some coconut milk for a swirly garnish.

mild cooking oil spray

1 medium onion, peeled and roughly chopped

2 garlic cloves, peeled and finely chopped

1tsp ground cumin

1tsp ground coriander

½tsp hot chilli powder

1 medium-large butternut squash (about 900g)

1 litre cold water

1 vegetable or chicken stock cube

400ml can reduced-fat coconut milk

fresh coriander, to serve

Makes 6 servings   **Ready in under 30 minutes**

1. Mist a large saucepan with the cooking oil and place over a low heat. Add the onion, garlic and spices. Cook gently for 8–10 minutes, stirring regularly until the onion is soft.

2. Peel the butternut squash and cut in half lengthways. Scoop out the seeds and discard. Cut the squash into roughly 2cm chunks. Pour the water into the pan with the onion and add the stock cube and butternut squash.

3. Bring to the boil, then reduce the heat slightly and simmer for a further 10 minutes, stirring occasionally until the squash is soft. Remove the pan from the heat and add the coconut milk. Blitz with a stick blender until smooth. (Puree the soup in a blender or food processor if you don't have a stick blender.)

4. Return to the hob and warm through gently without boiling, stirring and adding a little more water if the soup seems too thick. Serve hot, garnished with chopped fresh coriander if you have some handy.

Anna's Tip

This is a perfect 'slobbing in front of the telly' soup. Totally rich and totally satisfying.

Spicy Bean and Vegetable Soup

This soup is so filling that I sometimes have it as my evening meal served with a side portion of green beans or broccoli.

mild cooking oil spray

1 medium onion, peeled and finely chopped

2 garlic cloves, peeled and crushed

1–1½tsp hot chilli powder or smoked paprika

2 x 400g cans chopped tomatoes

400g can red kidney beans

400g can cannellini beans

1tbsp tomato puree

1 vegetable or chicken stock cube

1 red and 1 yellow pepper, deseeded

3 small courgettes, trimmed

198g can sweetcorn, drained

Makes 6 servings   **Ready in under 30 minutes**

1. Mist a large saucepan with the oil and gently fry the onion and garlic for about 5 minutes until very soft, stirring regularly. Stir in the chilli powder and cook for a further minute.

2. Tip the tomatoes into the pan, then refill the can with cold water and pour over the tomatoes. Drain and rinse all the beans. Add the beans, tomato puree and stock cube to the pan. Bring to a simmer and cook for 10 minutes, stirring occasionally.

3. Cut the peppers into roughly 1cm chunks. Cut the courgettes in half lengthways and then into 1cm slices. Stir the peppers into the pan and continue simmering for a further 5 minutes. Add the courgettes and sweetcorn.

4. Simmer the soup for 5 minutes more or until the courgettes are tender, stirring every now and then. Season with a little salt and some ground black pepper before serving.

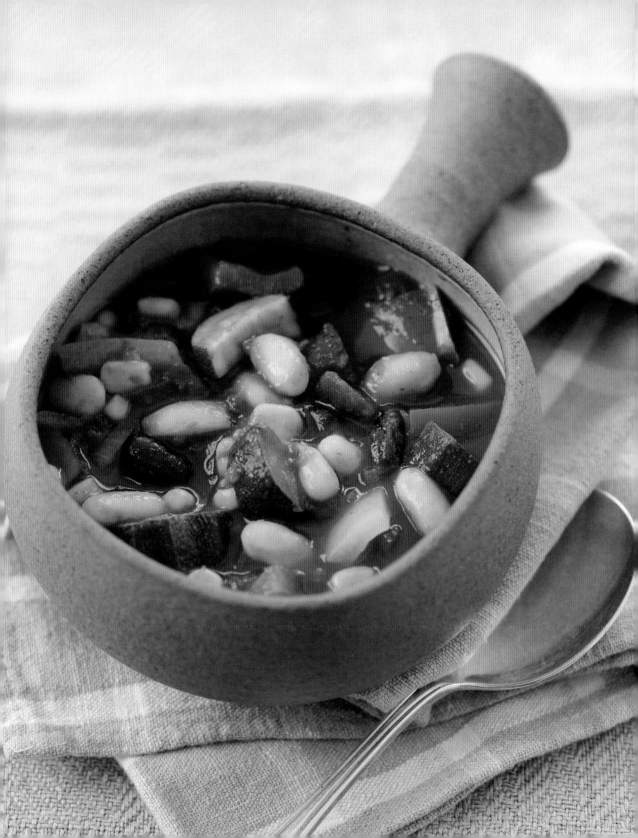

Salads

Whenever someone used to mention the word 'salad' I would immediately think of some wet iceberg lettuce, limp slices of cucumber and chunks of tomatoes that taste of nothing.

A recent trip to the States changed all of that for me, when I witnessed first hand just how ruddy fantastic a really great salad can be. So ruddy fantastic that I'll more often than not choose a salad from the menu, rather than having a hot meal, if I'm eating out.

I now tend to keep my fridge pretty well stocked with some wafer-thin ham, salmon, chicken or prawns. As long as I've got a bag of leaves, maybe a couple of tomatoes and some avocado, I can throw together a decent salad in no time.

Here you'll find some delicious main meal salads that can be served for lunch and loads that you can take to work if you want to. The ones without starchy carbs can be served in the evening too. Some are pretty basic, but there are also a few more exotic combinations, so why not give them a go?

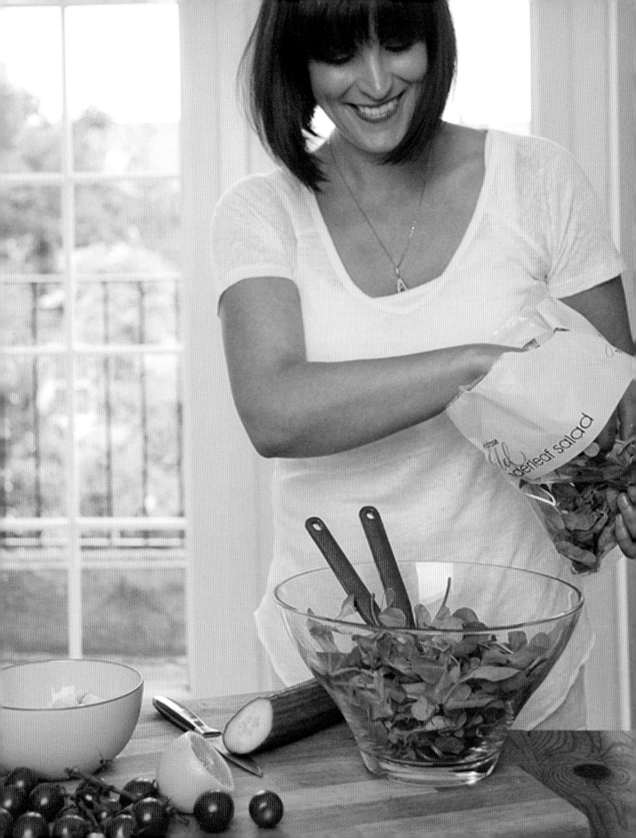

Smoked Mackerel Salad with Crunchy Croutons

I sometimes use peppered mackerel or hot-smoked salmon flakes for this salad. It's also a good one to put in the lunch box and take to work.

½ yellow pepper, deseeded

1 medium carrot, peeled

2 ripe tomatoes, quartered

a few slices of cucumber

1 celery stick, trimmed and thinly sliced

3–4 romaine lettuce leaves, roughly torn

1 smoked split mackerel fillet (roughly 50g), skinned

1 thin rye crispbread

1tsp hot horseradish sauce

1tsp salad cream

Serves 1   Ready in under 10 minutes

1. Cut the pepper and carrot into thin strips and put in a bowl with the tomatoes, cucumber, celery and lettuce leaves. Toss lightly together.

2. Flake the mackerel into chunky pieces and drop on top. Break the crispbread into small pieces and scatter over.

3. Mix the horseradish with the salad cream and 2tsp cold water in a small bowl. Spoon over the salad and serve.

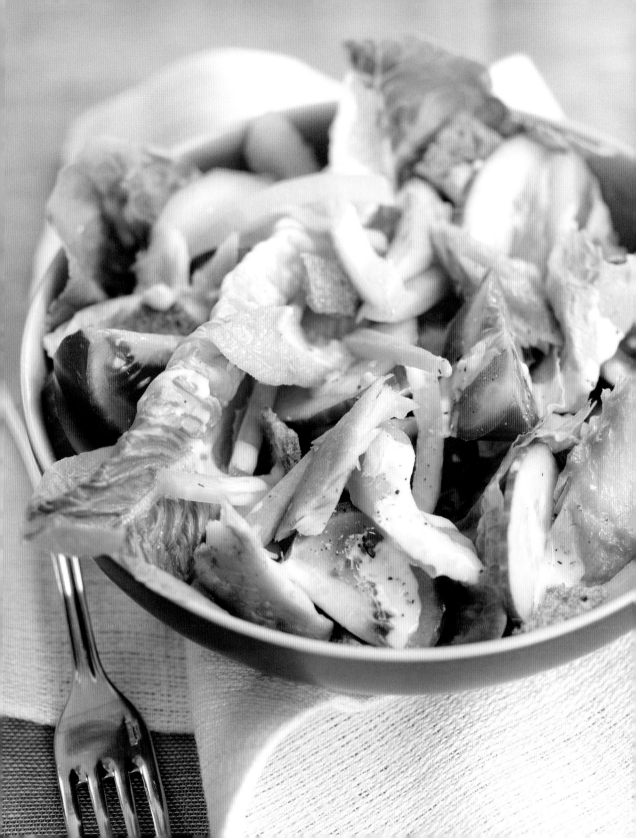

Tuna Niçoise

OK, so this Niçoise has no potatoes and the rich dressing is off the menu for the moment. It still tastes pretty damn good though, so give it a go...

2 medium
free-range eggs

large handful fine
green beans, trimmed

couple of handfuls
romaine lettuce leaves,
rinsed and drained

160g can tuna steak
in spring water or oil,
drained

6 canned anchovy
fillets in olive oil,
drained and halved
lengthways (optional)

4 ripe tomatoes,
quartered

handful black olives
(about 40g), drained

2–3tsp *Body Blitz*
dressing (page 61) or
balsamic vinegar

Serves 2   Ready in under 25 minutes

1. Half fill a small pan with water and bring to the boil. Gently place the eggs in the water and return to the boil. Cook for 9 minutes.

2. Drain the eggs in a colander and rinse under running water for a couple of minutes. Transfer to a large bowl of cold water and leave for at least 10 minutes until completely cold.

3. Meanwhile, half fill the pan with water again and bring to the boil. Cook the beans for 3–4 minutes until just tender, then drain and rinse under running water until cold.

4. Peel the eggs and cut into quarters. Roughly tear or shred the lettuce leaves and divide between two plates. Top with the eggs, beans, flaked tuna, anchovy fillets, tomatoes and olives.

5. Drizzle the dressing or a little balsamic vinegar over the salad and serve.

Spiced Fruity Chicken and Rice Salad

With the fruit, chicken and rice this is a really filling salad. Just add a few green leaves and you're done.

2tsp sunflower oil

½ medium onion, peeled and finely chopped

1tsp medium curry powder

1tbsp mango chutney

1tbsp tomato puree

100g (½ mug) easy cook long grain rice

1 ripe medium mango

1 apple, quartered, cored and sliced

handful seedless green grapes (100g), halved

1 skinless, boneless, cooked chicken breast, torn into pieces

small bunch fresh coriander, roughly chopped

lemon wedge, for squeezing

Serves 4   Ready in under 45 minutes

1. Heat the oil in a small non-stick frying pan and cook the onion for about 5 minutes until very soft. Stir in the curry powder and cook for a few seconds more, stirring constantly. Pour over 300ml cold water (about a mugful) and bring to the boil.

2. Stir in the mango chutney and tomato puree. Reduce the heat slightly and leave to simmer for 10 minutes or until all the liquid has reduced to around 6tbsp. Stir regularly, especially towards the end of the cooking time. Tip into a large mixing bowl. Leave until cold.

3. Half fill a medium pan with water and bring to the boil. Stir in the rice and return to the boil. Cook for 10 minutes or according to the packet instructions until tender. Rinse in a sieve under running water until cold. Drain well then tip into the bowl with the sauce.

4. Put the mango on a board and carefully cut down either side of the large, flat stone. Place, skin-side down, on the board and score through the mango flesh in a criss-cross fashion without cutting through the skin. Push the underside upwards with your thumbs and the mango pieces should separate. Use a small knife to scrape them off the skin into rice. Add the apple, grapes, chicken and coriander. Season with lemon juice and toss well.

Sweet Chilli Beef Salad

This dish is so simple but looks really impressive. And a touch of chilli sauce gives a sweet bite.

mild cooking oil spray

1 lean sirloin or rump steak (roughly 200g), trimmed of excess fat

2 medium carrots, peeled

½ small cucumber

1 small red pepper, deseeded

4 spring onions, trimmed

good handful each fresh coriander and mint leaves

FOR THE DRESSING

1tbsp sweet chilli dipping sauce

1tbsp sunflower oil

1tsp white wine vinegar

Serves 2   Ready in under 10 minutes

1. Heat a small non-stick frying pan over a high heat. Spray each side of the steak twice with oil. Season generously with freshly ground black pepper and place in the pan. Cook for 2 minutes on each side then transfer to a board and leave to rest for around 5 minutes.

2. Use a vegetable peeler to peel the carrot into thin ribbons, turning regularly. Do the same with the cucumber, discarding the central seedy part. Cut the pepper and spring onions into thin strips. Put all the vegetables in a bowl and scatter on the herbs.

3. To make the dressing, mix the dipping sauce and vinegar in a small bowl. Slice the steak lengthways into thin strips. Add to the bowl with the vegetables and toss together very lightly. Arrange on two plates. Spoon over the dressing, season with freshly ground black pepper and serve.

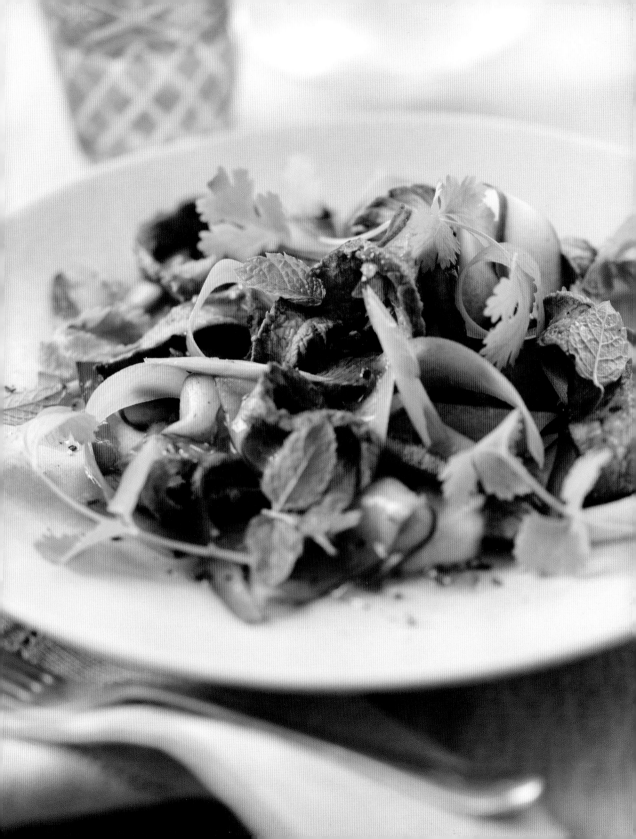

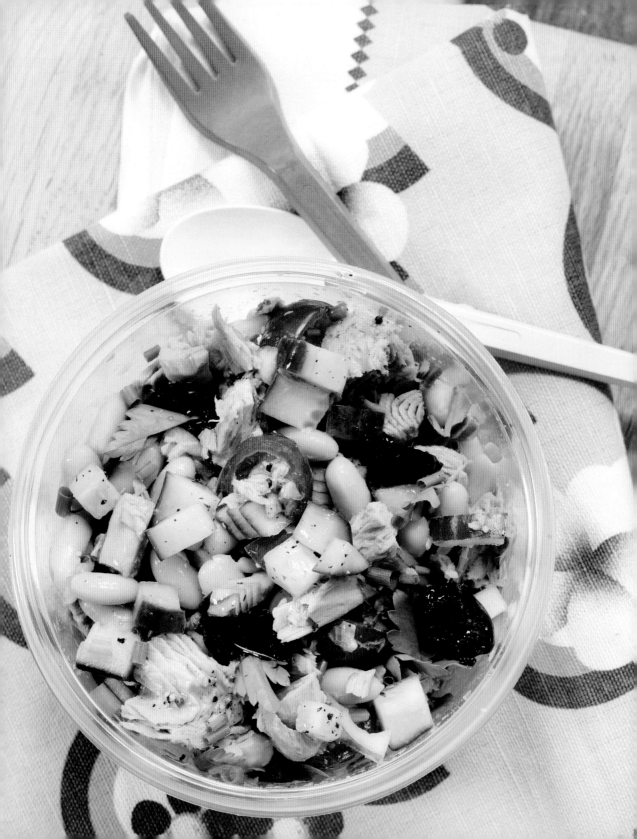

Tuna Bean Salad

This quick salad uses lots of storecupboard ingredients. The fresh herbs make it extra delicious but they're not essential. Put the rocket leaves on top and only mix when you're ready to serve the salad and they won't go limp.

160g can tuna steak in spring water or brine, drained

½ x 420g can cannellini beans, drained and rinsed

½ small red onion, peeled and diced

¼ cucumber, halved lengthways, deseeded and cut into roughly 1cm dice

6–8 pitted black or green olives, drained and halved (optional)

handful cherry tomatoes, halved

2tbsp roughly chopped flat leaf parsley (optional)

6–8 fresh chives, trimmed and finely sliced (optional)

freshly squeezed juice ½ lemon

1tbsp extra virgin olive oil

handful rocket or baby salad leaves (optional)

Serves 1   Ready in under 10 minutes

1. Tip the tuna into a bowl and flake into chunky pieces with a fork. Scatter the beans into the bowl and add the onion, cucumber, olives (if using), cherry tomatoes and herbs.

2. Stir the lemon juice and olive oil together in a small bowl and season with salt and pepper. Pour over the salad. Toss all the ingredients lightly and transfer to a small lidded container, leaving some space at the top if possible.

3. Put the salad leaves on top of the salad but do not mix until you are just about to serve. Keep cool. Either serve from the container or tip onto a plate.

Falafel Salad

Falafels make a great packed lunch, especially when combined with a spicy dressing. If you are making this recipe at home instead, warm the falafels before tossing into the salad.

handful baby gem lettuce leaves or torn romaine lettuce leaves

3–4 ready-made falafel balls

1 large carrot, peeled and cut into sticks

½ red pepper, deseeded and cut into sticks

¼ cucumber, cut into sticks

fresh mint and basil leaves (optional)

FOR THE DRESSING

½tsp harissa paste

1½tbsp mayonnaise

freshly squeezed lemon juice, to taste

Serves 1   Ready in under 10 minutes

1. Line a bowl or small, lidded container with the lettuce leaves. Add the falafel balls, vegetable sticks, mint and basil leaves, if using.

2. In a small bowl, mix the harissa paste and mayonnaise. Season with a little fresh lemon juice. Put into a tiny jam jar or little container and pack beside the salad. Cover the salad and dressing and keep cool.

3. When ready to serve, spoon the dressing over the salad.

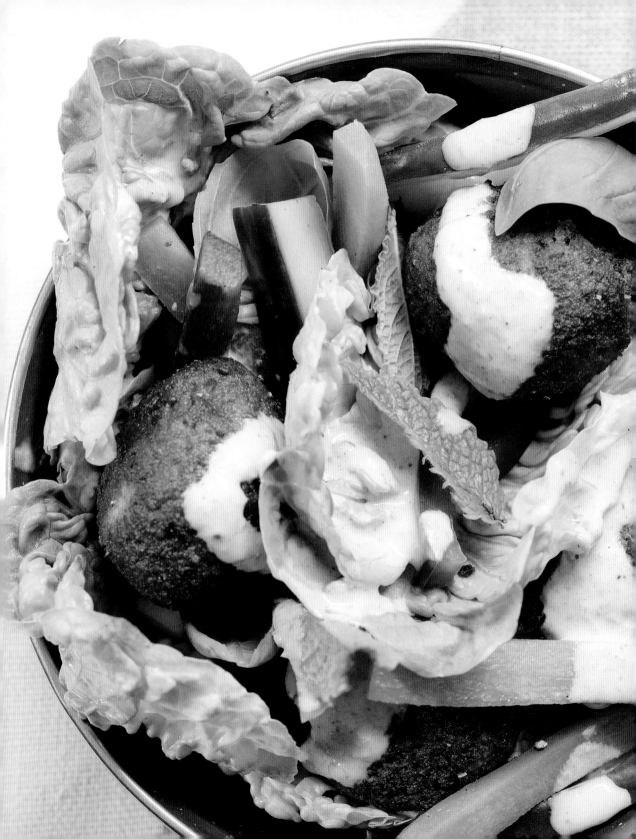

Dinners For Two

Watching your weight doesn't mean the death of your social life. We all want to spend time with the people we love, and guess what, you don't have to pile on the pounds to do it. These meal ideas are all easy, inspirational and impressive, and guaranteed to keep your other half happy too.

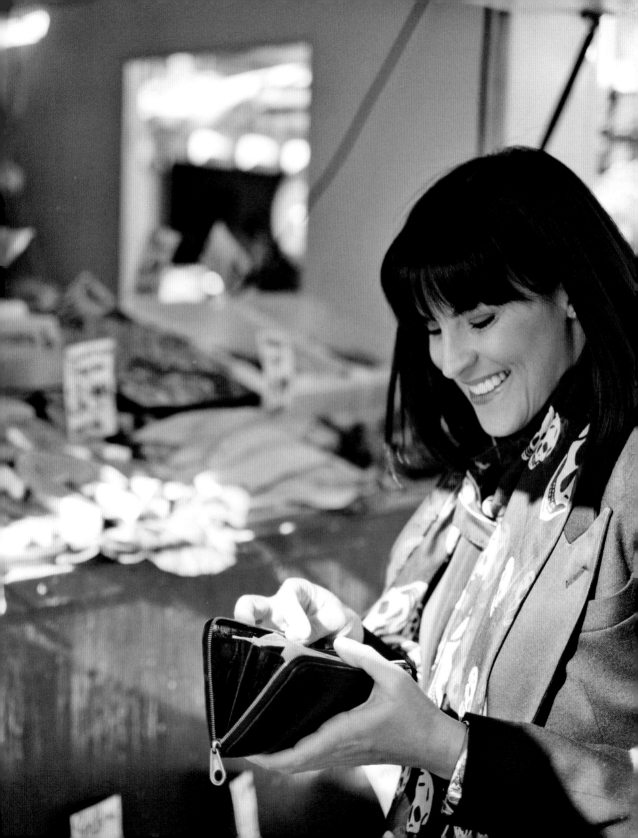

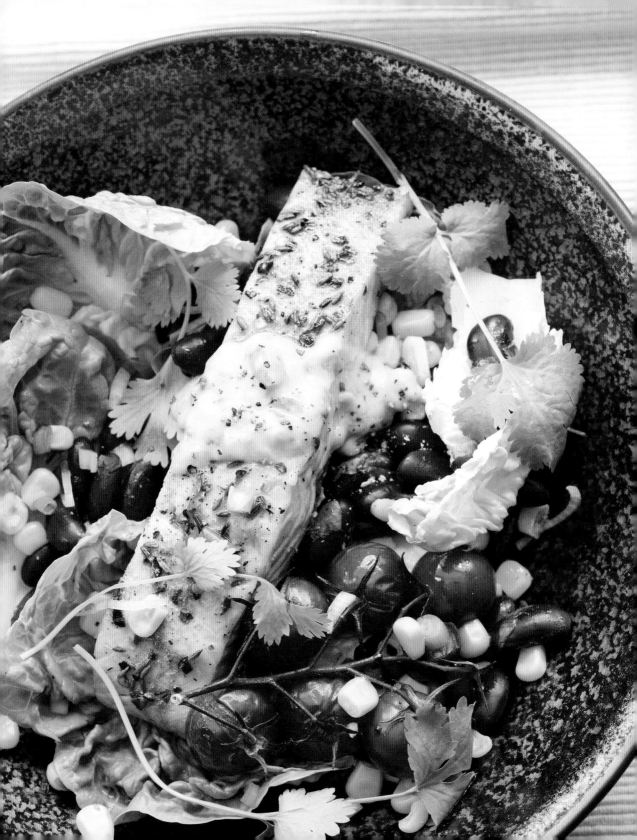

Mexican-Style Salmon

A filling and oh-so-healthy supper dish. If you are cooking for one, make the recipe for two and then use the leftover salmon and vegetables for a delicious salad the next day. If you don't fancy the salad this time, make the salmon according to the recipe and serve with mixed vegetables instead. Roasted vegetables go particularly well.

¼tsp dried chilli flakes

¼tsp cumin seeds

¼tsp ground coriander

2 x 125g plain or lightly smoked salmon fillets

mild cooking oil spray

2 vines cherry tomatoes, each with 6–7 tomatoes

FOR THE SAUCE

198g can sweetcorn, drained

200g canned red kidney beans, rinsed

4 spring onions, trimmed and sliced

small bunch fresh coriander, chopped

freshly squeezed juice ½ lime

1 small garlic clove, peeled and crushed

1tbsp olive oil

1 little gem lettuce, leaves separated

2tbsp ready-made salad dressing

Serves 2   Ready in under 30 minutes

1. Preheat the oven to 200°C/Gas 6. Mix the spices in a small bowl.

2. Place the salmon on a small foil-lined tin. Mist with a little oil, sprinkle with the spice mix and season with freshly ground black pepper and a little flaked sea salt. Add the cherry tomatoes to the tin. Bake the fish and tomatoes in the centre of the oven for 10–12 minutes.

3. While the salmon is cooking, mix the sweetcorn with the kidney beans, spring onions and coriander. Stir in the lime juice, garlic and olive oil. Season with a tiny pinch of salt and ground black pepper.

4. When the salmon is ready, remove from the oven and leave to stand for 3–4 minutes. Line two deep plates or bowls with the lettuce. Toss the bean salad quickly and spoon over. Add the tomatoes on their vines.

5. Put the salmon on top and spoon over a little dressing. Season with ground black pepper and serve while the salmon is warm.

Anna's Tip

If serving for one person, cook both salmon fillets but leave one to cool. Mix the beans with the dressing and put in a small, lidded container. Flake the salmon into large pieces on top and serve with little gem leaves and lemon wedges for squeezing. Keep cool.

Quick Prawn Balti

Juicy king prawns in a spicy tomato sauce – the perfect quick supper.

mild cooking oil spray

2tbsp medium or
balti curry paste

½ medium onion,
peeled and finely sliced

1tbsp mango chutney

4 ripe tomatoes,
quartered

200g (about 20) cooked
and peeled king prawns
(thawed)

100g pack (3–4 good
handfuls) baby
spinach leaves

Serves 2   Ready in under 15 minutes

1. Place a large non-stick frying pan or wok over a low heat and
mist with the cooking oil. Add the curry paste and onion. Cook
together over a medium heat for 3 minutes, stirring regularly
until the onion is softened.

2. Add the mango chutney, tomatoes and 200ml cold water.
Bring to a simmer. Leave to bubble for 4 minutes, stirring
occasionally until the tomatoes are soft but holding their shape
and the liquid has reduced by half.

3. Scatter over the prawns and spinach leaves. Stir-fry for 2–3
minutes or until the prawns are hot and the spinach is softened.
Serve in warm, deep bowls. (Add a small portion of rice if you're
having it for lunch.)

Anna's Tip

I love seafood and eat prawns all the time. But I'm also a big vegetarian food
fan, so try the veggie alternative – Quorn pieces – it works just as well.

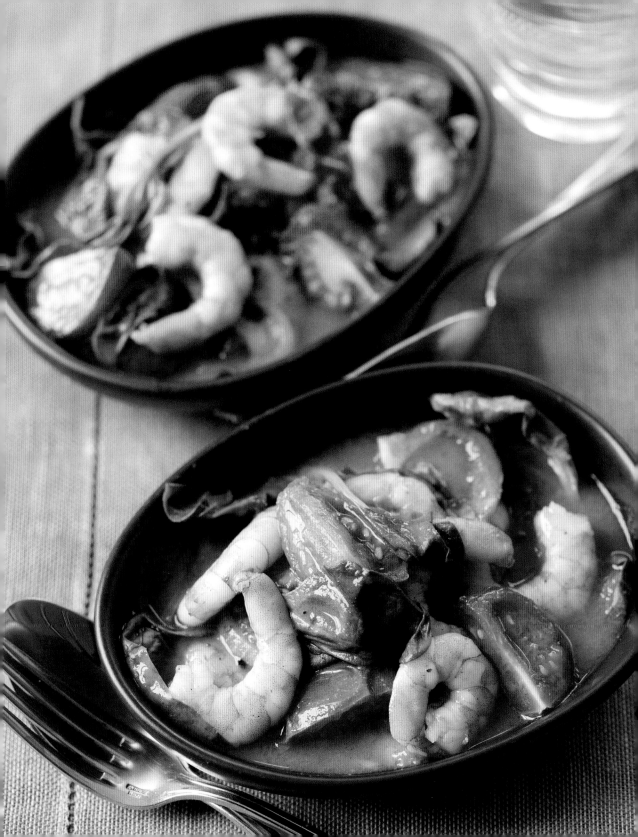

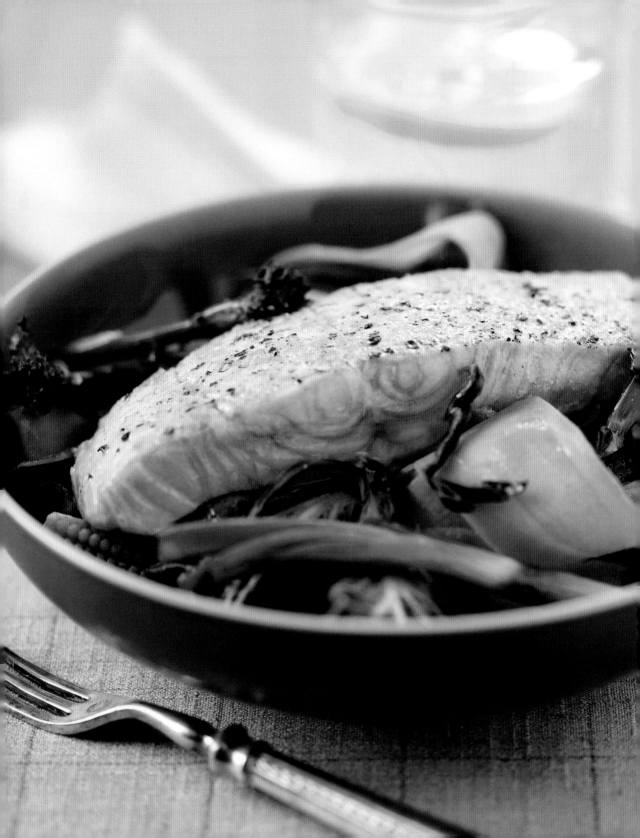

Pan-Fried Salmon with Stir-Fried Vegetables

How good does that salmon look? Go on – admit it – it looks great and only takes 15 minutes.

mild cooking oil spray

2 fresh salmon fillets (each about 125g with skin)

2tsp sunflower oil

1 packet (roughly 300g) fresh mixed stir-fry vegetables

dark soy sauce, to serve

Serves 2   Ready in under 15 minutes

1. Mist a large non-stick frying pan or wok with the cooking oil and place over a medium heat. Season the salmon generously with freshly ground black pepper.

2. Put the salmon in the pan, skin-side up, and cook for 4 minutes. Flip over and fry on the other side for a further 3–4 minutes or until just cooked. Lift the salmon carefully onto a small plate, cover loosely with foil and leave to stand while the vegetables are cooked.

3. Pour the oil into the frying pan or wok and add the vegetables. Stir-fry over a medium-high heat for 3–4 minutes, or according to the pack instructions, until just cooked. Sprinkle with a little soy sauce and toss well for a few seconds more.

4. Spoon vegetables onto serving plates and top with the hot salmon fillets. Serve immediately.

Anna's Tip

Even when I'm eating alone, I always cook 2 salmon fillets. The spare can be used in a salad the next day or for topping an open sandwich at lunch.

Saffron Fish Stew

I've always been too scared to cook a seafood stew because I don't know what to do. But Justine has made this dish so simple even I can do it.

500g very fresh live mussels

mild cooking oil spray

1 medium onion, peeled and finely sliced

2 large garlic cloves, peeled and finely sliced

freshly squeezed juice 2 large oranges (around 200ml)

a good pinch saffron threads

1tsp coriander seeds (optional)

2 bay leaves

6 ripe tomatoes, halved

300g skinless white fish fillet, such as cod or haddock, cut into large chunks

fresh coriander or parsley (optional)

Serves 2   Ready in under 25 minutes

1. Scrub the mussels really well and remove any beards. Discard any mussels with cracked or damaged shells or those that don't close when tapped on the edge of the sink. Rinse well.

2. Mist a large, deep non-stick frying pan or saucepan with cooking oil and gently fry the onion and garlic for 5 minutes, stirring regularly until softened but not coloured.

3. Pour the orange juice into the pan and add the saffron, coriander seeds, if using, bay leaves and tomatoes. Cover and simmer gently for 5 minutes or until the tomatoes are soft. Remove the lid and press the tomatoes with a wooden spoon to release the juice. Cook for 3 minutes more. Season with plenty of ground black pepper. Add a little extra water if your tomatoes aren't very juicy.

4. Stir in the mussels and the fish pieces. Cover tightly with a lid and steam over a high heat for 2–3 minutes until all the mussels have opened and the fish is just cooked (it should have turned completely white). Shake the pan a couple of times as the fish cooks.

5. Discard any mussels that don't open (and pick out the tomato skins if you want to). Sprinkle with finely chopped coriander or parsley if you have some and serve in deep bowls.

Anna's Tip

Use 200ml orange juice if you don't have fresh oranges to hand.

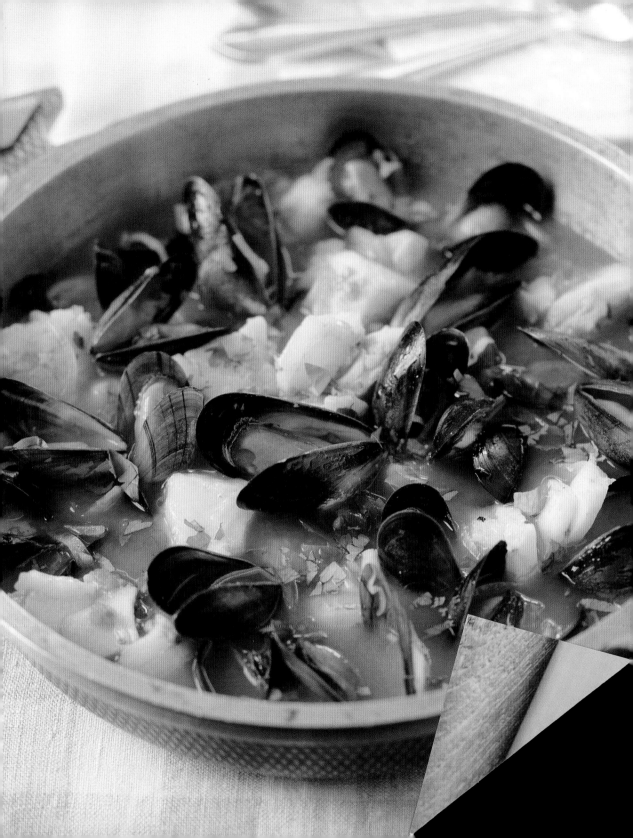

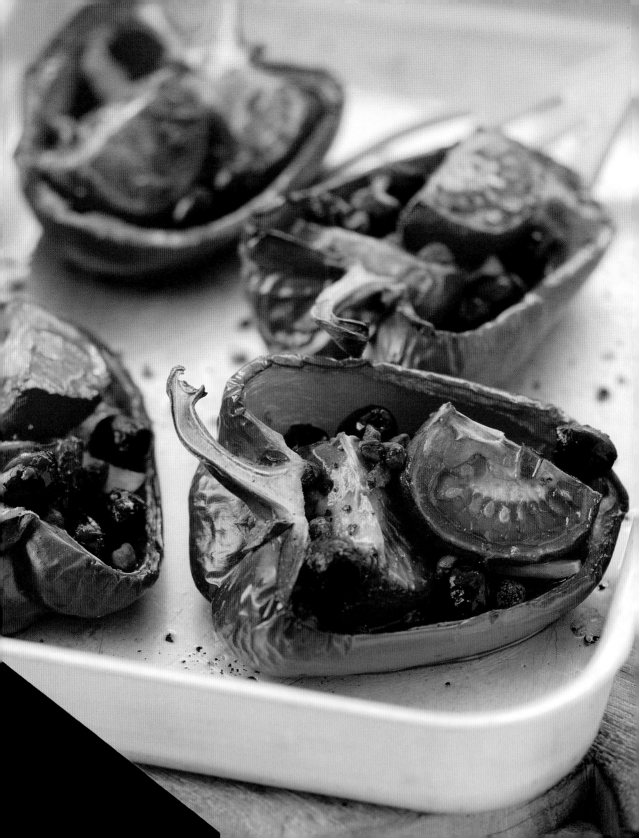

Roast Peppers with Olives and Capers

These peppers only take five minutes to prepare then you can put them in the oven and forget about them until you're ready to serve.

2 large red peppers, halved and deseeded

2 ripe tomatoes, quartered

1tbsp baby capers, drained

good handful small pitted black olives

1 large garlic clove, peeled and thinly sliced

1tsp extra virgin oil

handful fresh basil leaves (optional)

Serves 2   Ready in under 45 minutes

1. Preheat the oven to 200°C/Gas 6. Put the peppers, cut side up, in a small ovenproof dish or roasting tin. Place 2 tomato quarters inside each pepper half and divide the capers, olives and garlic between them.

2. Drizzle the peppers with the oil and season with plenty of freshly ground black pepper. Bake in the centre of the oven for 40 minutes.

3. Scatter the basil leaves over if you have some and serve with a lightly dressed salad or seasonal vegetables.

Anna's Tip

I like to bulk this dish out with other things to really fill me up. I'd either have a bowl of soup beforehand or a simple bean salad to go with it.

Five Minute Chilli and Coriander Prawns

These prawns make a great snack and taste great piled on top of a simple salad. Increase the quantities, poke a few cocktail sticks into them and you'll also have some delicious pre-dinner nibbles at your fingertips.

mild cooking oil spray

100g frozen raw peeled king prawns

finely grated zest ½ lime

1tbsp Thai sweet chilli dipping sauce

2tbsp roughly chopped fresh coriander leaves

freshly squeezed lime juice, to taste

Serves 1   Ready in under 5 minutes

1. Mist a small non-stick frying pan with oil and place over a medium heat. Stir-fry the prawns from frozen for 2 minutes (or thaw first if recommended on pack).

2. Add the lime zest, dipping sauce and coriander. Season with a touch of flaked sea salt and plenty of ground black pepper and stir-fry for a further 1–2 minutes or until completely pink and cooked throughout.

3. Remove from the heat, add a squeeze of lime juice to taste and serve hot or cold. (If serving cold, cool, cover and chill. Serve within 24 hours.)

Spicy Turkey Lettuce Wraps

This recipe is a little bit of fun and works as a perfect starter if you've got figure-conscious mates coming round.

thumb-sized chunk fresh root ginger

mild cooking oil spray

225g free-range turkey or chicken mince

6 spring onions, trimmed and finely sliced

1 plump red chilli, halved lengthways, deseeded and finely sliced

splash of soy sauce

6 romaine lettuce leaves, washed and drained

lime wedges, for squeezing

Serves 2   Ready in under 10 minutes

1. Peel and finely grate the root ginger, discarding the fibrous bits (you'll need about 2tbsp). Set aside. Mist a large non-stick frying pan or wok with the cooking oil and place over a high heat. Add the turkey or chicken mince and cook for 3 minutes, constantly using 2 wooden spoons to break up the clumps.

2. Stir the ginger, spring onions and chilli into the pan and fry with the mince for a further minute or until the turkey or chicken is cooked – it should be completely white with no pink remaining. Sprinkle over the soy sauce and toss through the mince. Tip into a bowl.

3. To serve, scoop the hot mince mixture into the lettuce leaves and squeeze over a little lime juice. Eat with fingers.

Anna's Tip

These wraps are so light that you can follow them with a mango and strawberry fruit salad if you like. Serve half a mango and a handful of strawberries per person.

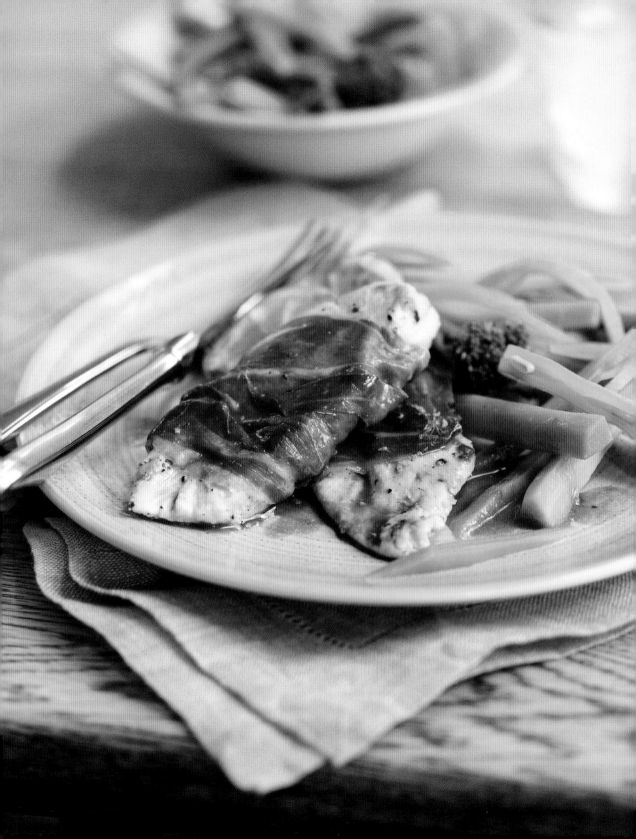

Lemony Chicken Wrapped in Parma Ham

Another great supper recipe, perfect for cooking quickly after a hard day at work.

2 skinless, boneless, free-range chicken breasts

freshly squeezed juice 1 small lemon

4 slices Parma ham

mild cooking oil spray

knob of sunflower or olive oil spread

3tbsp water

Serves 2   Ready in under 10 minutes

1. Put the chicken breasts on a chopping board and very carefully slice horizontally through the middle and open out into two halves.

2. Sprinkle half the lemon juice over the chicken. Season on both sides with a little salt and plenty of freshly ground black pepper. Wrap each chicken piece in Parma ham.

3. Mist a small non-stick frying pan with the oil and place over a medium-high heat. As soon as the pan is hot, fry the chicken on each side for about 3 minutes or until cooked through. Transfer the chicken to two warmed plates.

4. Drop a knob of sunflower or olive oil spread into the pan and as soon as it melts, pour over the remaining lemon juice and water and stir together for a few seconds until the sauce is smooth. Pour over the chicken and serve.

Anna's Tip

This is a great dish for summer or winter. If the weather is cold, I'll have mountains of steamed vegetables and in the summer, just slice it up and scatter on some salad leaves.

Moroccan-Style Chicken

Chicken is a dieter's best friend but it can be difficult to make it interesting, especially if you are new to cooking like me. I've learned that by adding just a few simple spices you can transform the bland into the beautiful.

½tsp ground coriander

½tsp ground cumin

½tsp dried chilli flakes

finely grated zest of
½ lemon or lime

2 boneless, skinless
free-range chicken
breasts

mild cooking oil spray

Serves 2   Ready in under 25 minutes

1. Preheat the oven to 200°C/Gas 6. Mix all the spices in a small bowl with the grated lemon or lime zest, a good pinch of salt and a few twists of freshly ground black pepper.

2. Carefully slash the top of each chicken breast diagonally 5 times with a sharp knife. Sprinkle with the mixed spices and rub in well.

3. Mist a small baking tray with cooking oil and put the chicken breasts on top. Spray with a little more oil.

4. Bake in the centre of the oven for 18–22 minutes or until thoroughly cooked. (The chicken should be white in the middle with no pink remaining.)

5. Take out of the oven and leave to stand for 3–4 minutes. Cut into thick diagonal slices and serve with a salad of fresh mint leaves and tomatoes. Add a small portion of barley couscous if you are having it for lunch.

Anna's Tip

Add some quartered lime to the tin and roast alongside the chicken. Squeeze over to serve.

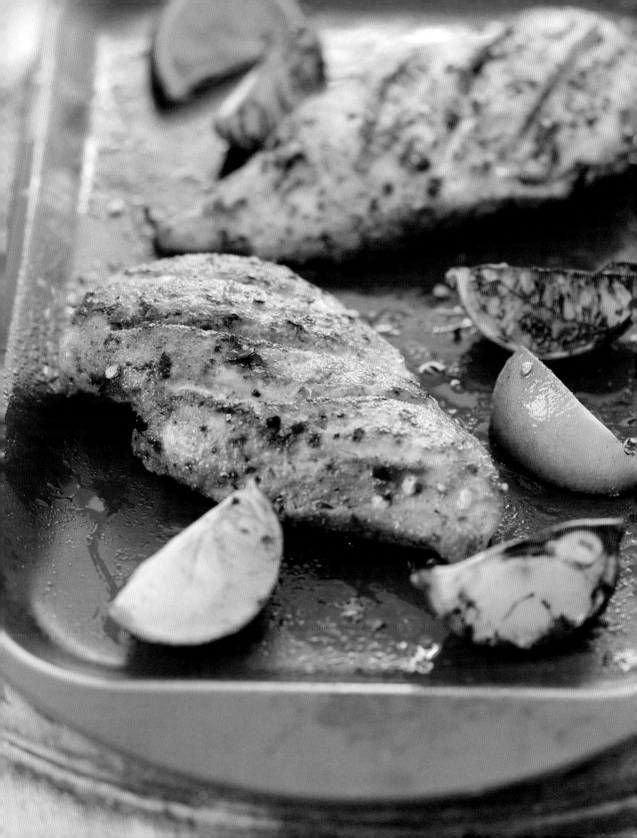

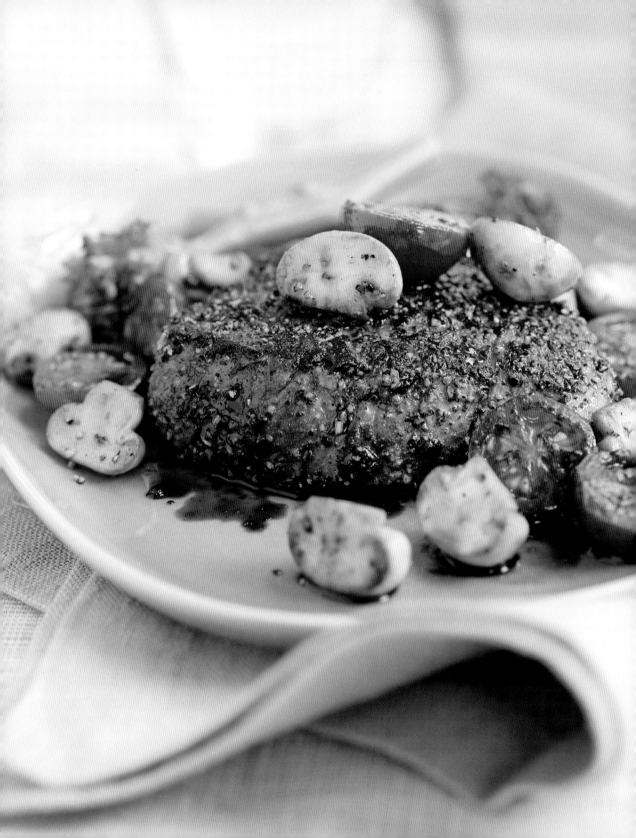

Peppered Steak with Mushrooms

A juicy pan-fried steak with mushrooms is the ultimate 'I can't believe I'm on a diet' dinner for two.

2 fillet or thick rump steaks (about 150g each), trimmed of excess fat

mild cooking oil spray

couple of handfuls button mushrooms, wiped and halved

handful cherry tomatoes, halved

splash balsamic vinegar or Worcestershire sauce

Serves 2   Ready in under 10 minutes

1. Coat the steaks really well on both sides with coarsely ground black pepper and a little salt. Mist a small non-stick pan with the cooking oil and place over a medium-high heat.

2. When the pan is hot, add the steaks and cook for 4 minutes on each side for medium rare. Increase the cooking time by roughly a minute each side for medium steak and 2 minutes if you like it well done.

3. Transfer the steaks to 2 warmed plates. Tip the mushrooms into the pan and spray a few times with the cooking oil. Stir-fry for 2 minutes until softened and beginning to colour. Keep the pan hot or they will stew rather than fry.

4. Add the cherry tomatoes to the pan and cook with the mushrooms for 1 minute more, turning regularly until the tomatoes soften. Remove from the heat and season with a splash of balsamic vinegar or Worcestershire sauce. Spoon over steaks and serve.

Anna's Tip

If you're cooking for 1, fry up an extra steak, chill overnight and slice into a salad the next day.

Herb-Rubbed Rack of Lamb with Butter Bean Mash

This elegant dinner is perfect for a special occasion.

2tbsp finely chopped thyme leaves or 2tsp dried thyme

2tbsp finely chopped mint leaves or 2tsp dried mint

½tsp flaked sea salt

1 rack well-trimmed lamb (with 6–7 ribs)

mild cooking oil spray

200ml lamb stock (made with 1/3 stock cube)

2tsp good balsamic vinegar

FOR THE BUTTER BEAN MASH

400g can butter beans, drained

1 garlic clove, peeled and crushed

1 sprig rosemary

1tsp freshly squeezed lemon juice

Serves 2   Ready in under 25 minutes

1. Preheat the oven to 200°C/Gas 6. Mix the herbs with the salt and plenty of freshly ground black pepper in a bowl. Put the lamb on a board and rub all over with the herb mixture.

2. Mist a small non-stick frying pan with the cooking oil and place over a medium-high heat. Put the lamb in the pan and cook for 2–3 minutes on each side until lightly browned, turning carefully with tongs.

3. Transfer the lamb to a small baking tray and finish cooking in the oven for a further 10 minutes (if you prefer your lamb well done, add an extra 5 minutes). Return the frying pan to the hob and stir in the lamb stock and balsamic vinegar. Bring to the boil and cook for 2–3 minutes until the sauce is reduced to just 3–4tbsp.

4. Remove the lamb, transfer to a plate and leave to rest for 5 minutes. Meanwhile, blend the butter beans and garlic with 4tbsp cold water in a food processor. Scrape into a saucepan, add the rosemary and lemon juice. Season with salt and pepper and heat through gently, stirring regularly until hot.

5. Carve the lamb into cutlets. Spoon the mash onto 2 warmed plates, discarding the rosemary. Place the lamb on top and spoon over the sauce. Serve with freshly cooked vegetables.

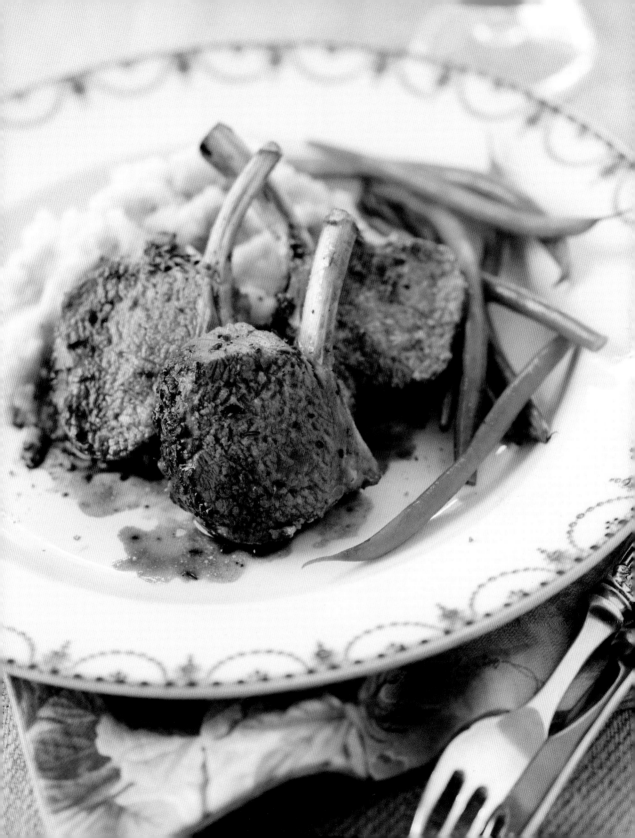

Dinners in a Dash

Stuck for time or inspiration? Try some of these simple suppers and serve with a huge salad or loads of freshly cooked vegetables. They are all designed to serve one, but just increase the quantities for more servings. And don't forget, if you increase the quantities, you'll need to increase the cooking times too.

• Lemon and Black Pepper Chicken

Put 1 boneless, skinless free-range chicken breast in a small baking tray lined with foil and slash three times with a knife. Bring up the edges of the foil a little. Pour over the juice of 1 lemon. Season with lots of freshly ground black pepper. Drizzle with 2tsp olive oil. Bake in a preheated oven at 200°C/Gas 6 for 18–22 minutes or until the chicken is cooked.

• Warm Chicken Salad

Place 1 boneless, skinless free-range chicken breast between 2 sheets of cling film and bash with a rolling pin until around 1cm thick. Mist a small non-stick frying pan with mild cooking oil. Season the chicken with salt and pepper. Fry for 5 minutes on each side over a medium-high heat until browned and cooked through. Tear leaves from ½ romaine lettuce heart and put on a plate with a handful of cherry tomatoes, halved. Drizzle with 1tbsp *Body Blitz* dressing.

• Chicken with Chilli and Lime

Put 1 boneless, skinless free-range chicken breast in a small baking tray lined with foil. Bring up the edges of the foil a little. Drizzle with 2tsp olive oil. Pour over the juice of 1 lime. Sprinkle with ½tsp dried chilli flakes mixed with the zest of 1 lime. Season with a little salt and pepper. Bake in a preheated oven at 200°C/Gas 6 for 18–22 minutes or until the chicken is cooked.

• Chickpeas with Cumin, Spinach and Tomatoes

Heat 1tbsp olive oil in a large non-stick frying pan. Gently fry ½ small onion, finely sliced, and 1 garlic clove, crushed, for 5 minutes until well softened. Stir in 1tsp each ground cumin and ground coriander. Cook for 1 minute, stirring. Add ½ x 400g can drained chickpeas and 2 medium tomatoes, roughly chopped. Stir-fry for 3 minutes then add 2 big handfuls baby spinach leaves and a squeeze of lemon. Cook for a further 2–3 minutes, stirring. Season with plenty of ground black pepper.

• Balsamic Salmon

Mist a small ovenproof dish with mild cooking oil. Place 3 sliced spring onions in the dish. Put 1 x 150g fresh salmon fillet on top and place 6 whole cherry tomatoes around it. Drizzle with 1tbsp balsamic vinegar. Bake in a preheated oven at 200°C/Gas 6 for 12–15 minutes until cooked.

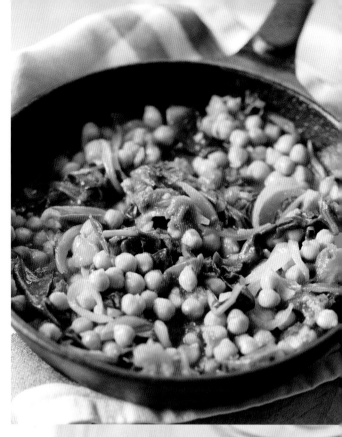

• Baked Fish with Tomato and Basil

Mist a small ovenproof dish with mild cooking oil. Place 1 x 200g thick white fish fillet, such as cod or haddock, in the dish. Spread with 2 heaped tbsp tomato and basil stir-through pasta sauce. Bake in a preheated oven at 200°C/Gas 6 for 18–20 minutes or until cooked through. Sprinkle with fresh basil leaves to serve.

• Minted Lamb Burger

Mix 125g lean minced lamb with 1 shallot, finely chopped and 2tsp mint sauce. Season. Form into a burger shape. Mist a small non-stick pan with mild cooking oil spray. Fry the burger over a medium heat for about 5 minutes on each side or until nicely browned and cooked through.

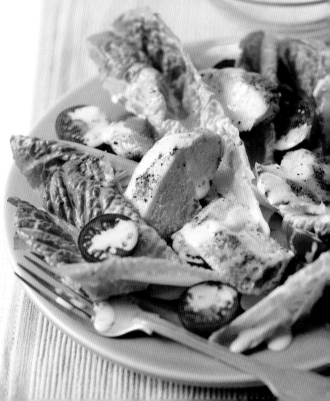

Family Food

When you have a family to feed dieting can be a total nightmare. So many people have told me that they don't want to have to cook two different dishes every time the family sits down together.

This section is specifically designed for healthy eating that the whole family can enjoy. We've got some recipes here that even the fussiest of eaters will find hard to resist.

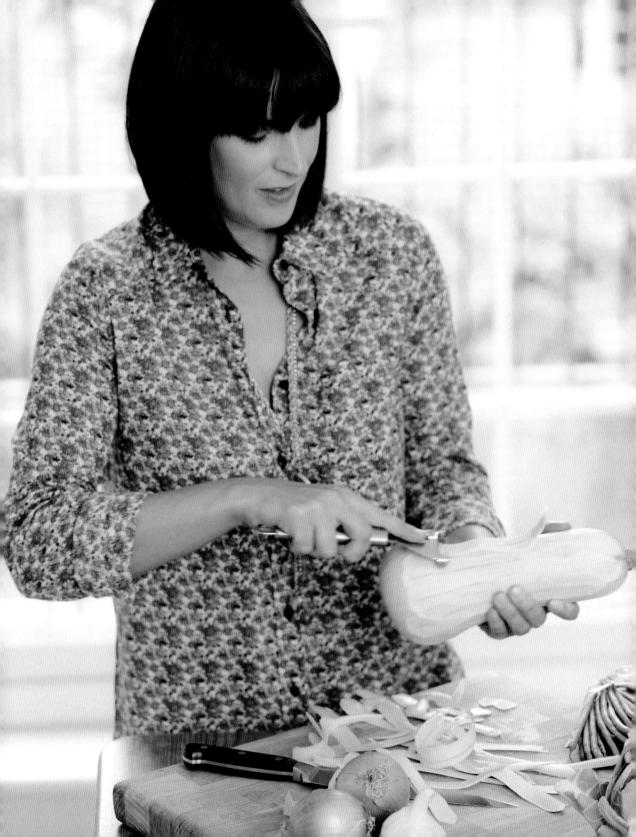

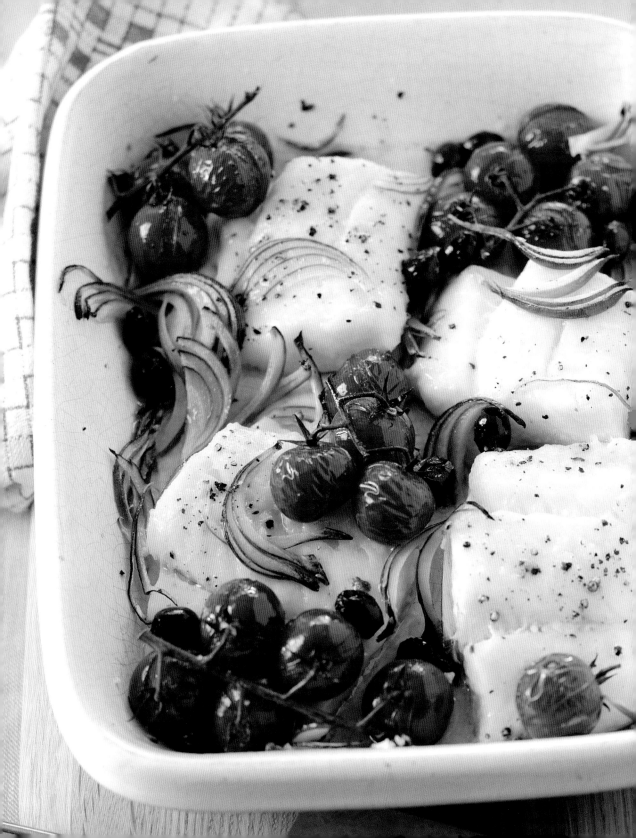

Baked Fish with Tomatoes and Olives

I make this with any thick white fish fillets – cod and haddock both work well. Try to choose fish from sustainable sources and do a bit for the environment as well as your waistline.

4 fresh, thick white fish fillets (about 175g each), skinned

4 short vines cherry tomatoes

a good handful (50–75g) small pitted black olives, drained

1 medium red onion, peeled and cut into thin wedges

2tbsp extra virgin olive oil

Serves 4   Ready in under 20 minutes

1. Preheat the oven to 200°C/Gas 6. Put the fish in a shallow, ovenproof dish with the tomatoes. Scatter the olives and onion over. Season with plenty of freshly ground black pepper and, little salt. Drizzle with olive oil.

2. Bake in the centre of the oven for 18–20 minutes or until the fish is cooked and the tomatoes are softened. You can test the fish by inserting a knife into the centre of 1 of the fillets – it should look completely white inside.

3. Serve with heaps of freshly cooked vegetables or a large, lightly dressed salad.

Anna's Tip

I use all sorts of different olives for this dish, whichever I have in the cupboard or buy at the deli counter work really well.

Spatchcock Jerk Chicken

Spatchcocking a chicken is loads easier than you might imagine – all you need is a really strong pair of scissors. If in doubt, you can always ask your butcher to do it for you. This zesty marinade is packed with Caribbean flavour and goes down a treat when you've got a few mates round.

1.5kg free-range chicken

freshly squeezed juice 1 lime

1 tsp sunflower oil

1 tbsp jerk seasoning

finely grated zest 1 lime

3tbsp chopped fresh thyme leaves

Serves 4–6   Ready in under 1 hour, plus marinating

1. To spatchcock the chicken, put the chicken on a board, breast-side down. Using a strong kitchen scissors, poultry shears or a large, sharp knife, cut very carefully from the tail end each side of the spine to the neck, cutting through the rib bones as you go.

2. When you have removed the backbone, turn the chicken over and flatten it with your hands until around the same thickness all over. Rub the chicken with the lime juice and then the oil. Slash through the thickest part of each breast 3–4 times.

3. Mix the jerk seasoning in a bowl with the lime zest and the chopped thyme. Rub the seasoning all over the chicken. Place on a large plate or tray and cover with cling film. Leave to marinate in the fridge for a few hours until you need it.

4. Transfer the chicken to a roasting tin. Roast in a preheated oven at 200°C/Gas 6 for 35–40 minutes, ensuring the chicken is cooked through and no longer pink before serving. (Alternatively, barbecue the chicken over a medium-high heat for 20 minutes on each side or until thoroughly cooked.)

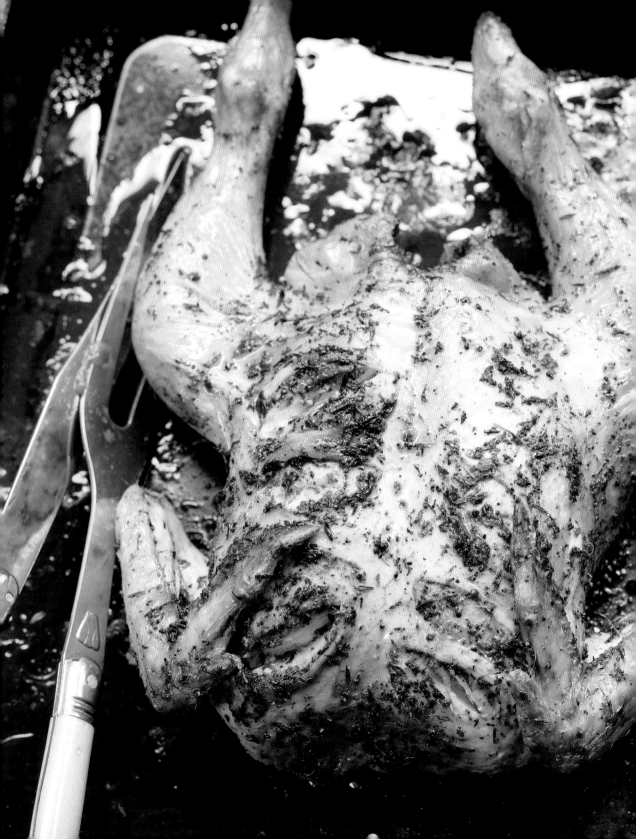

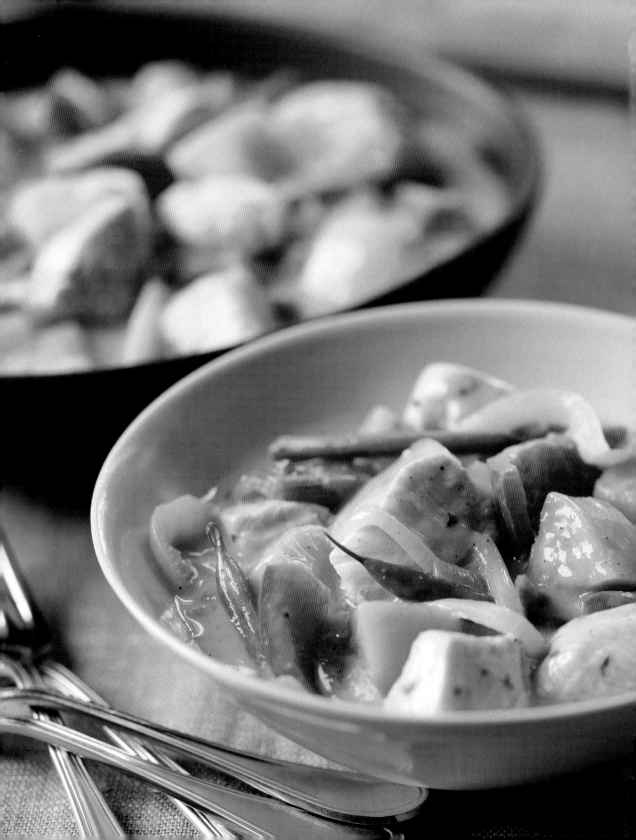

Creamy Chicken Curry

I'm a big fan of curry and spicy dishes so it's great to know that I can still indulge without piling on the pounds.

½ small butternut squash (400g), peeled and deseeded

3 free-range boneless, skinless chicken breasts

1 red and 1 yellow pepper, deseeded

a handful (100g) green beans

2tbsp medium curry or balti paste

1 medium onion, peeled, halved and sliced

400ml can reduced-fat coconut milk

1tbsp cornflour mixed with 2tbsp cold water

freshly chopped coriander, to serve (optional)

Serves 4   Ready in under 30 minutes

1. Cut the butternut squash into roughly 2cm chunks and the chicken and peppers into roughly 3cm chunks. Cut the beans in half. Put the curry paste in a large, non-stick saucepan. Add the onion and squash and cook over a medium heat for 2–3 minutes, stirring.

2. Pour over the coconut milk and half fill the can with cold water. Pour into the pan and bring to a simmer. Cook the onion and squash for 5 minutes, stirring occasionally.

3. Add the chicken, peppers and beans. Return to a simmer and cook for a further 8–10 minutes or until the chicken is cooked through and the vegetables are tender, stirring occasionally.

4. Stir the blended cornflour into the curry sauce. Cook for 1–2 minutes more, stirring until thickened. Serve hot, sprinkled with a little freshly chopped coriander if you have some.

Anna's Tip

Serve with freshly cooked rice or warm naan bread for the rest of the family – but make sure you keep your hands off!

Lemon Roasted Chicken

I love a traditional roast and there's no reason not to enjoy this one just because you're watching your weight. Just make sure you eat your chicken without the skin and serve with lots of freshly cooked vegetables.

1 free-range roasting chicken (about 1.5kg)

½ large lemon

1 medium onion, peeled, halved and sliced

4 rashers rindless dry-cure (preferably) back bacon

2tsp cornflour mixed with 1tbsp cold water

Serves 4 (with leftovers) Ready in under 1¾ hours

1. Preheat the oven to 190°C/Gas 5. Remove any elastic that may be trussing the chicken. Put the chicken on a board and squeeze the lemon juice all over. Rub the lemon juice into the chicken skin and season with flaked sea salt and black pepper.

2. Put the onion in a pile in the centre of a sturdy roasting tin and place the chicken on top. Don't allow too much onion to escape around the chicken as it may burn. Pop the squeezed lemon half inside the chicken. Roast in the centre of the oven for 45 minutes per 1kg, plus 20 minutes. (Around 1½ hours.)

3. Half an hour before the end of the cooking time, carefully remove the chicken from the oven and cover with bacon rashers. Return to the oven until the chicken is thoroughly cooked. The juices should run clear when the thigh is pierced with a skewer.

4. Transfer the chicken and bacon to a warmed serving dish and scoop up any onions that you are able to lift from the pan and place beside it. Leave to rest. Holding the pan carefully with an oven cloth, tilt all the juices to one corner. Skim as much fat from the surface as possible and discard.

5. Put the roasting tin on the hob over a low heat and add 200ml cold water. Stir well to lift the juices and sediment from the bottom of the pan – these will add heaps of flavour to the gravy. Carefully transfer to a medium saucepan and bring to a simmer. Stir in the cornflour mixture. Cook for 1–2 minutes until thickened, stirring constantly. Serve with carved chicken, onions and bacon.

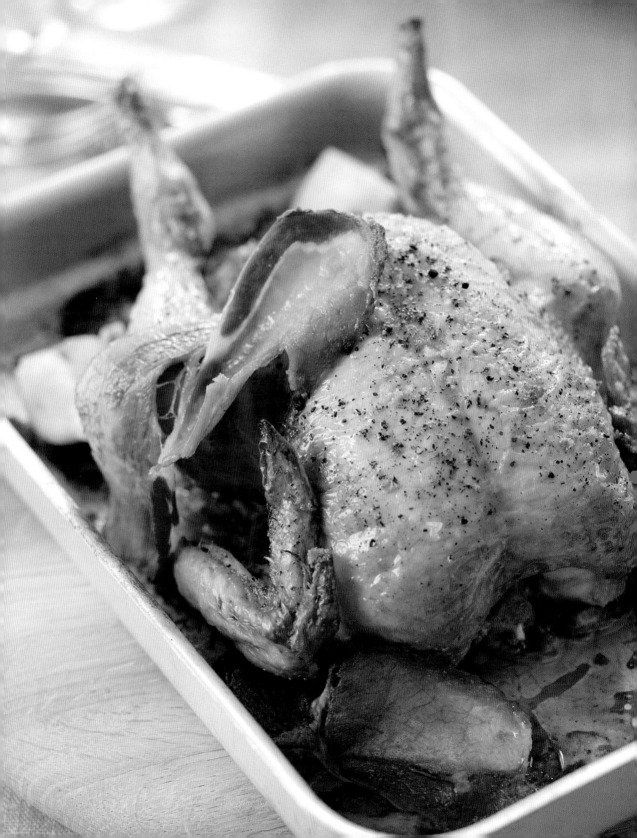

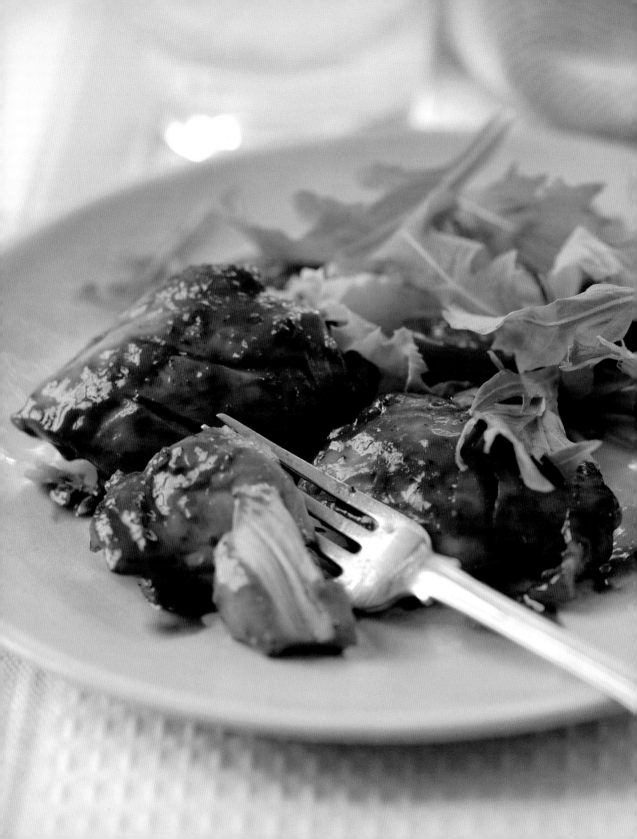

Sticky Chicken Thighs

Take a look at the photo to the left. Does it look like diet food?
No. And it doesn't taste like it either.

4tbsp tomato ketchup

2tbsp Worcestershire sauce

1tbsp Caribbean-style hot pepper sauce

6 boneless, skinless free-range chicken thigh fillets

Serves 2–3   Ready in under 40 minutes

1. Preheat the oven to 200°C/Gas 6. Put the ketchup, Worcestershire and pepper sauces in a small bowl and mix well.

2. Slash the top of each chicken thigh diagonally 2–3 times with a knife and place in a small ovenproof dish. (It should fit pretty snugly in one layer.)

3. Spoon over the sauce mixture and turn the chicken a couple of times until well coated. Bake for 30 minutes or until the chicken is completely cooked.

4. Remove the dish and transfer the chicken to a plate. Holding the dish with an oven cloth, carefully pour the sauce into a medium saucepan and bring to the boil. Cook for about 3–4 minutes, stirring regularly until the sauce is thick.

5. Place the chicken in the pan and turn to coat in the sticky sauce. Heat through for a minute or so. Serve with a large, lightly dressed salad or lots of vegetables.

Homemade Burgers

Juicy, meaty homemade burgers are very easy to make – even for me. These ones have some grated carrot in the mix that helps them keep deliciously moist.

500g lean minced beef

1 medium onion, peeled and coarsely grated or finely chopped

1 large carrot, peeled and finely grated

2 garlic cloves, peeled and finely chopped

1 heaped tsp dried mixed herbs

mild cooking oil spray

large crunchy salad and 1tbsp mayonnaise per person, to serve

Serves 6   Ready in under 20 minutes

1. Put the mince in a large bowl with the onion, carrot, garlic and herbs. Add a good pinch of salt and plenty of freshly ground black pepper.

2. Mix until well combined – you can use your hands for this bit if you like. Form the mixture into 6 balls and flatten into burger shapes.

3. Mist a large non-stick frying pan with the cooking oil and fry the burgers gently for 5–6 minutes on each side until nicely browned and cooked throughout.

4. Serve with a colourful, crunchy salad, topped with a little mayonnaise or ketchup.

Anna's Tip

For summer barbecues, I like to spice these burgers up a bit. Just add 1tsp each dried chilli flakes, ground cumin and ground coriander with 1tbsp tomato puree to the burger mix and see how different they taste.

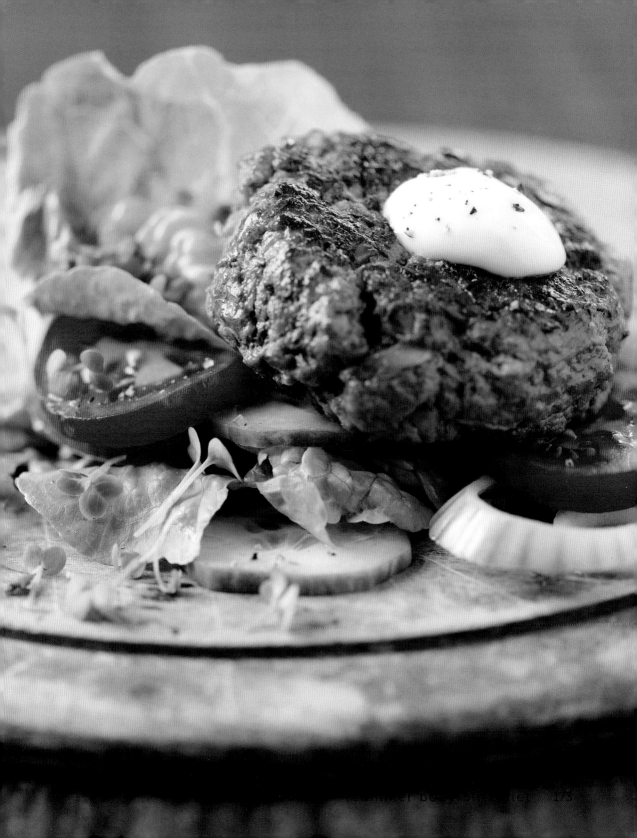

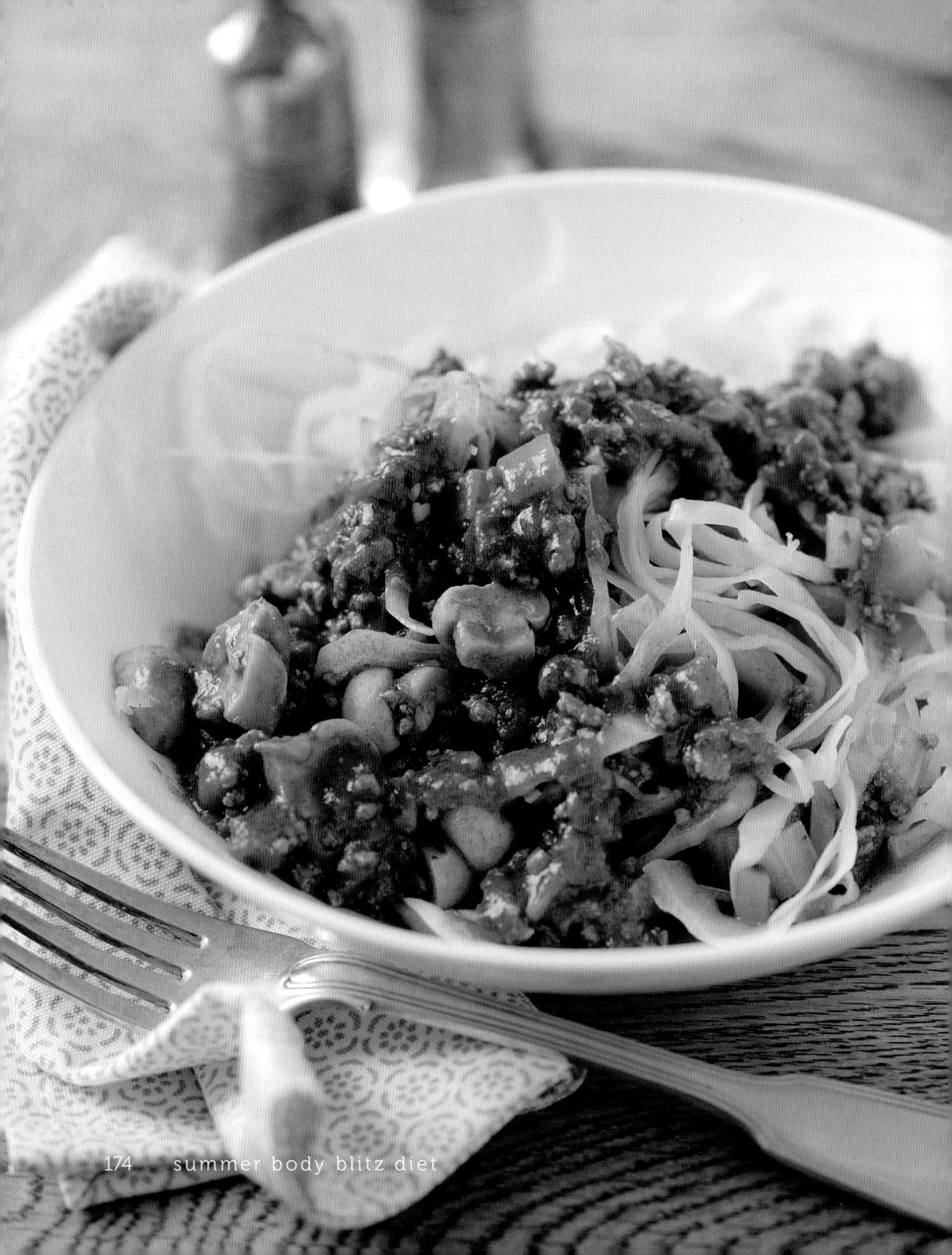

Bolognese Sauce

Instead of serving your Bolognese with fattening pasta, spoon it on top of lightly boiled, finely shredded cabbage – Cheat's Spaghetti! A vegetable serving and no starchy carbs, but you'll hardly notice the difference.

500g lean minced beef

1 medium onion, peeled and finely chopped

2 sticks celery, trimmed and finely sliced

2 medium carrots, peeled and finely diced

2 garlic cloves, peeled and crushed

couple of handfuls (roughly 100g) button mushrooms, wiped and halved

400g can chopped tomatoes with herbs

2tbsp tomato puree

1 beef stock cube

1tbsp cornflour

Serves 4–6   Ready in under 1 hour

1. Fry the mince with the onion, celery, carrots and garlic in a large non-stick saucepan over a medium heat for 5 minutes or until the beef is no longer pink. Stir the meat with a wooden spoon to break up any large clumps.

2. Add the mushrooms and fry with the mince and vegetables for a further 2–3 minutes. Stir in the tomatoes and tomato puree. Refill the tomato can with cold water and pour into the pan. Crumble the stock cube over the top, season with ground black pepper, give a good stir and bring to a simmer.

3. When the liquid is bubbling, but not too madly, cover the pan loosely with a lid and leave to simmer over a low heat for 35 minutes, stirring occasionally. Mix the cornflour with 1tbsp cold water in a small bowl and stir into the pan 2–3 minutes before the end of the cooking time. Simmer until thickened. Season to taste with salt and pepper.

Mini Cottage Pies with Parsnip and Apple Mash

These cute little pies are popular with kids and can be made well ahead of time.

500g lean minced beef

1 medium onion, peeled and finely chopped

2 sticks celery, trimmed and finely sliced

2 medium carrots, peeled and finely diced

2 garlic cloves, peeled and finely chopped

400g can chopped tomatoes with herbs

2tbsp tomato puree

1 beef stock cube

1tbsp cornflour

FOR THE MASH

4 medium parsnips, peeled and cut into small chunks

1 large Bramley apple, peeled, quartered, cored and cut into small chunks

small knob of sunflower or olive oil spread

splash of semi-skimmed milk

Serves 6   Ready in 1¼ hours

1. Fry the mince with the onion, celery, carrots and garlic in a large non-stick saucepan over a medium heat for 5 minutes or until the beef is no longer pink.

2. Add in the tomatoes and tomato puree. Refill the tomato can with cold water and pour into the pan. Crumble the stock cube over the top, season with a few twists of ground black pepper, give a good stir and bring to a simmer.

3. When the liquid is bubbling, but not too madly, cover the pan loosely with a lid and leave to simmer gently over a low heat for 35 minutes, stirring occasionally. Mix the cornflour with 1tbsp cold water in a small bowl and stir into the pan. Cook for 2 minutes.

4. While the mince is cooking, prepare the mash. Half fill a medium pan with cold water and bring to the boil. Add the parsnips and cook for 15 minutes. Add the apple chunks and cook for a further 5 minutes until tender. Preheat the oven to 200°C/Gas 6.

5. Drain the parsnips and apple in a colander, then return to the saucepan and add the sunflower or olive oil spread, milk, a little sea salt and plenty of ground black pepper. Mash until as smooth as possible.

6. Spoon the mince mixture into 6 individual pie dishes or one large ovenproof dish. Top with the mash. Put on a baking tray and cook for about 20 minutes.

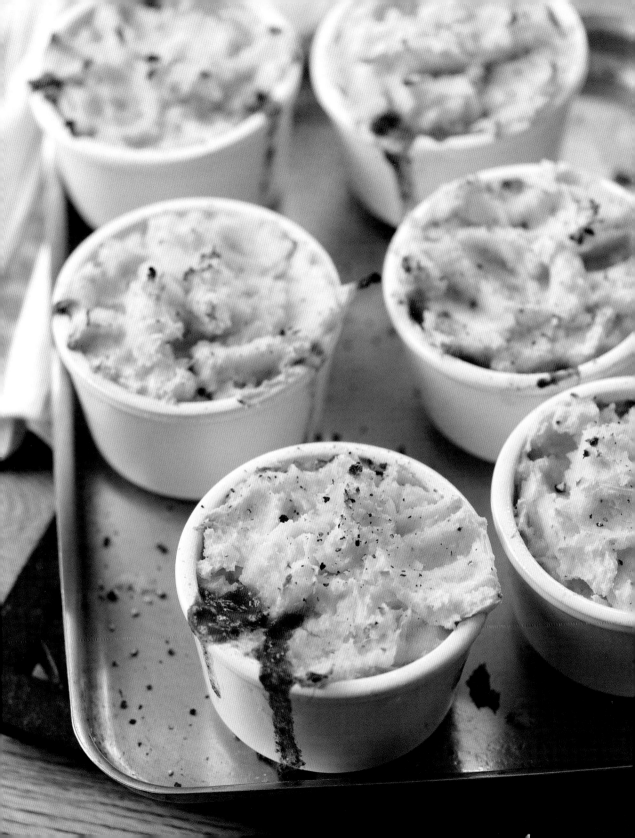

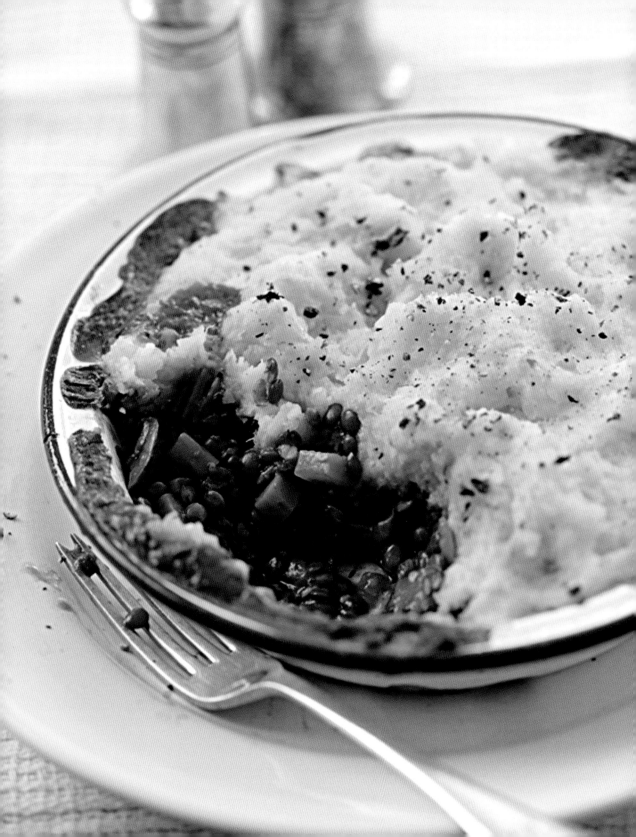

Gardener's Pie

I'm a big fan of healthy, filling vegetarian pies. Instead of traditional mash, use celeriac or parsnips.

1tbsp sunflower oil

1 small onion, peeled and finely chopped

1 garlic clove, peeled and finely chopped

2 medium carrots, peeled and diced

2 sticks celery, trimmed and diced

large handful small chestnut mushrooms, wiped and sliced

100g puy lentils (roughly ½ mug), rinsed

400g can chopped tomatoes with herbs

1 vegetable stock cube

2tsp tomato puree

1tbsp cornflour mixed with 1tbsp cold water

FOR THE TOPPING

1kg celeriac, peeled and cut into roughly 2cm pieces

small knob sunflower or olive oil spread

Serves 4   Ready in under 1 hour

1. Mist a large non-stick saucepan with the oil and gently fry the onion, garlic, carrots and celery for 5 minutes or until beginning to soften, stirring regularly. Add the mushrooms to the pan and cook for 2 minutes over a high heat until lightly browned, stirring.

2. Add the lentils and tomatoes. Refill the tomato can with cold water twice and pour into the pan. Add the crumbled stock cube and tomato puree. Bring to the boil, then reduce the heat slightly and simmer for 30 minutes or until the lentils are tender, stirring occasionally. Add a little extra water if necessary.

3. Meanwhile, half fill a medium saucepan with water and bring to the boil. Add the celeriac and return to the boil. Cook for 12–15 minutes or until very tender. Preheat the oven to 220°C/ Gas 7. Drain the celeriac well in a colander then return to the saucepan and mash with the sunflower or olive oil spread and a little salt and plenty of freshly ground black pepper. Set aside.

4. When the lentils are tender, add the cornflour mixture and cook for 1–2 minutes more, stirring until the sauce thickens. Spoon into a 1-litre ovenproof dish. Top with the mash, working around the edge of the dish before heading into the middle.

5. Place the dish on a baking tray and cook in the centre of the oven for 20 minutes or until the topping is pale golden brown and the filling is bubbling. Serve with lots of freshly cooked green vegetables.

Meatballs in Tomato Sauce

Meatballs are a real family favourite and there's no reason why you can't enjoy them too. I've used grated courgette instead of breadcrumbs to keep these ones really juicy.

300g lean minced beef

1 small onion, peeled and finely chopped

2 garlic cloves, peeled and crushed

1 medium courgette, trimmed and finely grated

1tsp dried mixed herbs

mild cooking oil spray

500g jar tomato pasta sauce

Serves 4   **Ready in under 30 minutes**

1. Put the mince in a large bowl with the onion, garlic, courgette and herbs. Add a good pinch of salt and plenty of freshly ground black pepper. Mix until well combined – you can use your hands for this bit if you like. Form the mixture into 16 small balls.

2. Mist a large, deep non-stick frying pan or saucepan with the cooking oil and fry the meatballs gently for 5 minutes, turning regularly until nicely browned on all sides. Carefully drain off any fat that has collected in the pan..

3. Stir the pasta sauce into the frying pan, then half fill the jar with cold water and stir into the sauce. Bring to a gentle simmer and cook for 20 minutes, stirring occasionally until the meatballs are tender and the sauce is thickened. Serve with tagliatelle for the family and a large, crunchy salad for you.

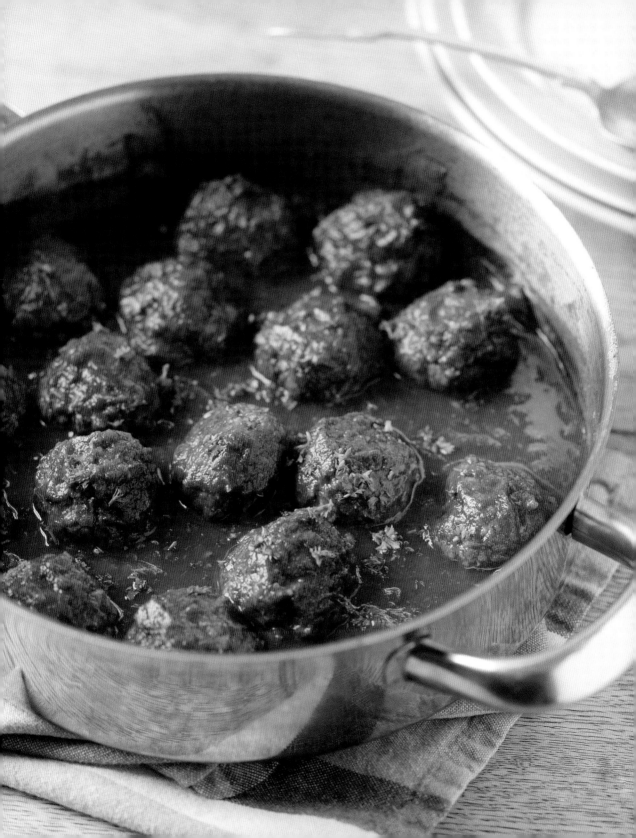

Roast Pork with Baked Apples

Instead of roasting potatoes around your pork, add a few small apples and use apple juice instead of wine to add flavour to the gravy and a delicious fruity tang.

1.2–1.4kg rolled loin of pork

6 small apples, cut in half

200ml fresh pressed apple juice

5 fresh sage leaves, finely chopped or a good pinch dried sage

2tsp cornflour

a few fresh sage leaves, to garnish (optional)

Serves 6   Ready in under 2 hours 10 minutes

1. Preheat the oven to 180°C/Gas 4. Place the pork in a small, sturdy roasting tin. Roast for 35 minutes per 500g, plus 35 minutes. (A 1.2kg joint will take 2 hours.) Half an hour before the end of the cooking time, remove the tin and place the apples around the pork. Return to the oven to finish cooking.

2. When the pork is cooked, transfer to a platter with the apples, cover loosely with foil and leave to rest. Holding the pan carefully with an oven cloth, tilt all the juices to one corner. Skim as much fat from the surface as possible and discard.

3. Put the roasting tin on the hob over a medium heat and add the apple juice, fresh or dried sage and 50ml cold water. Stir well to lift the juices and sediment from the bottom of the pan – these will add heaps of flavour to the gravy. Simmer for a couple of minutes.

4. Carefully strain the gravy into a medium saucepan and bring to a simmer. Mix the cornflour with 1tbsp cold water and stir into the gravy. Cook for 1–2 minutes until thickened, stirring constantly. Carve the pork and serve yourself up to three slices (without crackling!), two apple halves, a couple of spoonfuls of the gravy and plenty of freshly cooked vegetables.

Sausages with Onion Gravy

Choose really meaty wheat-free pork sausages for this quick recipe. If you're having it for your evening meal, avoid sausages containing rice.

mild cooking oil spray

8 good-quality wheat-free pork sausages

1 medium onion, peeled, halved and thinly sliced

250ml beef stock made with ½ beef stock cube

1tbsp tomato ketchup

2tsp cornflour

Serves 4   Ready in under 20 minutes

1. Lightly mist a large non-stick frying pan with cooking oil and fry the sausages over a medium heat for 5 minutes, turning occasionally.

2. Add the onion to the pan and cook with the sausages for a further 5 minutes or until the sausages are cooked through and the onions are softened and golden brown. Transfer the sausages to a plate and stir the stock and ketchup into the frying pan.

3. Mix the cornflour with 1tbsp cold water in a small bowl until smooth. Stir into the onion mixture. Bring to a simmer and cook until thickened, stirring. Return the sausages to the pan and reheat in the hot gravy for a minute or 2. Serve with lots of freshly cooked vegetables.

Anna's Tip

I like making this recipe using vegetarian sausages and I serve them with loads of freshly cooked vegetables.

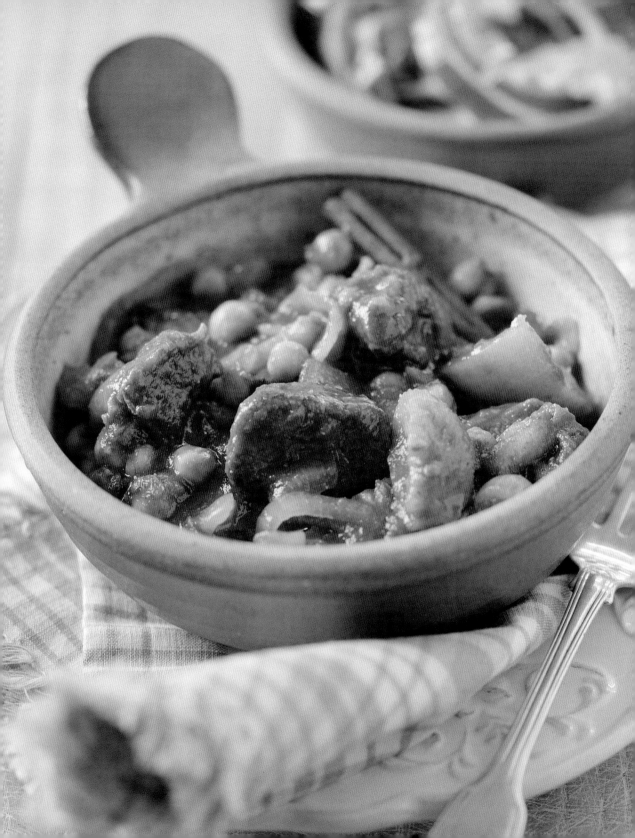

Fruity Lamb Tagine

Tender lamb in a spicy sauce with chickpeas and tomatoes makes a perfect meal to serve for friends. Don't worry about browning the meat and you'll cut the fat and the calories – but no one will notice.

800g lean lamb leg meat

1 large onion, peeled, halved and sliced

2 garlic cloves, peeled and finely chopped

1tsp each ground cumin, and ground coriander

½–1tsp hot chilli powder

good pinch saffron threads

2 cinnamon sticks

400g can chickpeas, rinsed and drained

12 no-soak dried apricots, quartered

½ small lemon, quartered

400g can chopped tomatoes

Serves 6   Ready in under 2 hours

1. Preheat the oven to 180°C/Gas 4. Cut the lamb into roughly 3cm chunks. Put the lamb, onion, garlic, all the spices, chickpeas, apricots and lemon in a large flameproof casserole. Add the tomatoes, then refill the can with cold water twice and pour over the other ingredients. Stir well.

2. Place the casserole over a medium heat and bring slowly to the boil. Remove from the heat and cover with a lid. Carefully transfer to the oven. Cook for 1½ hours or until the lamb is tender. Stir halfway through the cooking time. Serve with a large salad or lots of green beans.

Anna's Tip

If you don't want to use lamb for this recipe, swap for boneless, skinless, chicken thighs or a small butternut squash, peeled, deseeded and cut into chunks. Cook for 45 minutes.

Lamb Koftas with a Minty Cucumber Salad

Lamb koftas make a great alternative to burgers. Choose the leanest lamb mince you can find. They're delicious served hot and almost as nice cold.

500g lean minced lamb

1 medium onion, peeled and finely chopped

2 garlic cloves, peeled and finely chopped

finely grated zest 1 lemon

1tsp ground cumin

1tsp ground coriander

½tsp chilli powder

¼tsp ground cinnamon

3tbsp finely chopped fresh mint leaves

FOR THE CUCUMBER SALAD:

½ large cucumber cut into small dice

handful fresh mint leaves, finely chopped

1–2tsp freshly squeezed lemon juice

1tbsp extra virgin olive oil

Serves 6   Ready in under 25 minutes

1. Mix the lamb mince in a large bowl with the onion, garlic, lemon zest, spices, mint, a good pinch of flaked sea salt and plenty of freshly ground black pepper until well combined. Form the meat mixture into 18 balls or shape into ovals if you prefer.

2. To grill the koftas, thread onto long metal skewers. Place on a foil-lined baking tray under a medium-high grill and cook for 3–4 minutes on each side or until no longer pink in the middle.

3. To oven bake, place on a foil-lined baking tray and cook in a preheated oven at 200°C/Gas 6 for 15 minutes or until no longer pink in the middle, turning once .

4. To fry the koftas, mist a non-stick frying pan with oil spray and place over medium heat. Cook the koftas for 8–12 minutes, turning occasionally until well browned and cooked throughout.

5. For the cucumber salad, mix the cucumber with the mint, lemon juice, olive oil, a pinch of salt and some ground black pepper. Serve with the hot koftas and a large mixed salad.

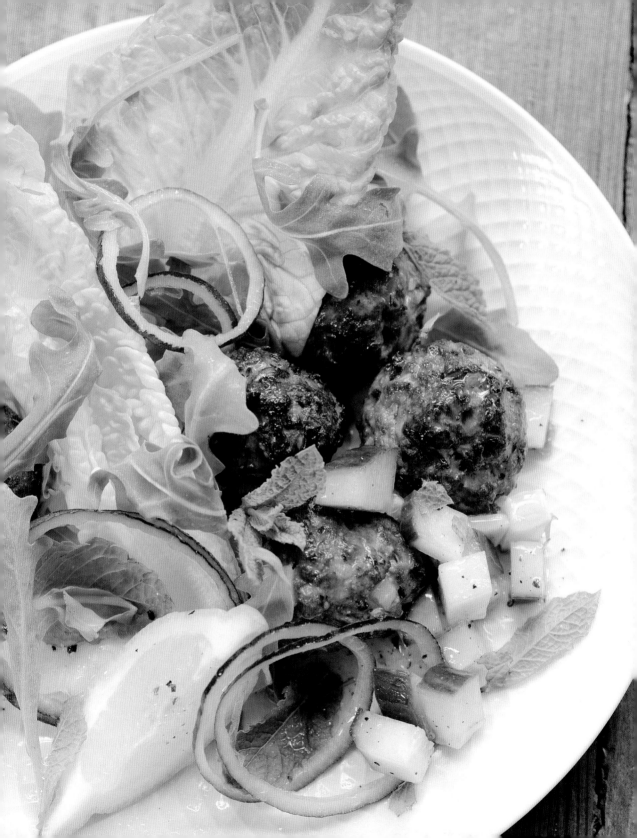

Quick Fixes

When I'm manically busy at work or even just lazing at the weekend, I don't really feel like going to the effort to make a full meal for myself. But I know I'm hungry and I need to eat something quick – without resorting to the takeaway menu or legging it down to the corner shop. This is when Quick Fixes are so useful.

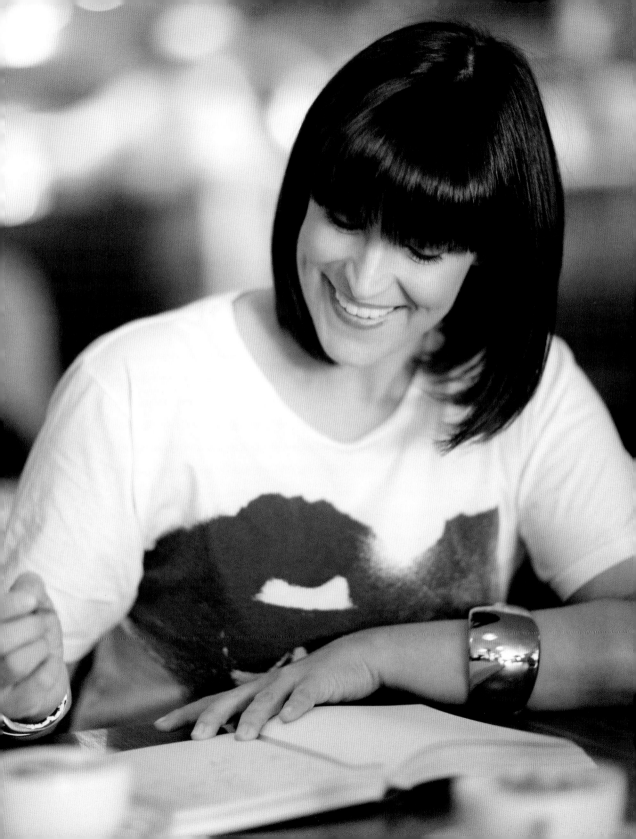

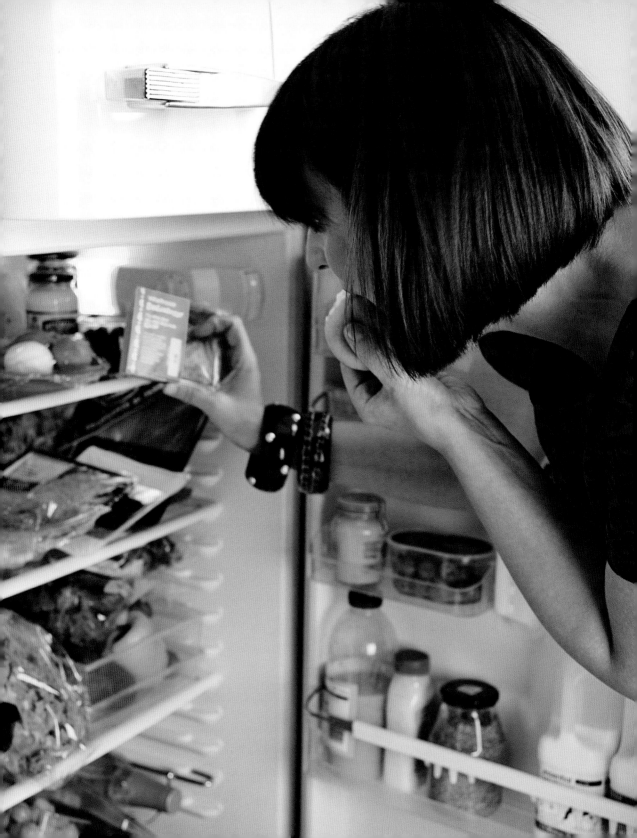

Fast Food

I reckon that people often fail when losing weight because the pressure to eat something completely different each day is incredibly difficult for most of us. Don't get me wrong, I like to eat different things – I just don't necessarily want, or need to every day. With this in mind, we've devised a way for you to have a huge variety of foods with very little hassle.

Quick Fix food is always in my house – whether stashed in the fridge or the cupboards. It's the sort of stuff that's really easy to throw together but tastes great and, more importantly, adheres to **The Rules**.

Quick Fix food is perfect for anyone with a busy lifestyle because there's always something you can grab for lunch or dinner. **Quick Fix** food is also perfect for meals on the go as all the ingredients are fully prepared and only need chucking in a packed lunch box.

I also try and serve my **Quick Fixes** with a simple salad of some kind. And, as always, only have the carbs with your lunch – never dinner.

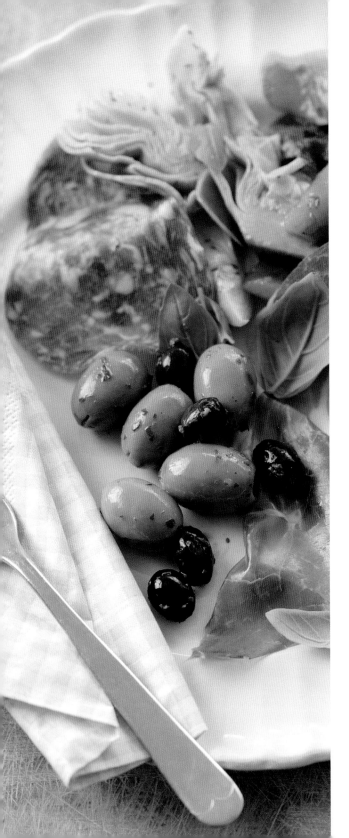

Take Five

For any meal, you need to pick five items. They can be a combination of five completely different things, or maybe two servings of one item, like ham for instance, plus three of any others. If there's something you'd like that isn't on the list, feel free to eat it as long as it conforms to **The Rules.** Remember – be sensible about your portion size! You can make the foods as exotic or as simple as you like. **Here are two of my favourites:**

● Deli Platter

Handful olives, any kind – green or black, marinated, stuffed or plain

8 pieces (75g) char-grilled peppers, drained

4 char-grilled baby artichokes, drained

2 slices Parma ham

3 slices salami

rocket salad with cherry tomatoes

● English Salad

3 slices lean ham

1 large free-range egg, hard-boiled

1tbsp salad cream

½ slice rye bread, spread thinly with sunflower or olive oil spread

baby gem lettuce, cucumber, celery and grated carrot

Your Quick Fix Platter

Choose **FIVE items** from any of the following lists and add a salad.

• Meats

3 slices (50g) lean ham

8 slices (50g) wafer-thin ham

2 slices (30g) Parma ham or prosciutto

3 thin slices (20g) salami or chorizo

2 slices (40g) cold roast chicken or turkey

2 small slices (30g) cold roast beef or pork

½ small skinless roast chicken breast (40g)

• Fish and Seafood

2 slices (40g) smoked salmon

1 smoked trout fillet (40g)

35g roasted or poached salmon

15g split smoked mackerel fillet

6 marinated white anchovies (30g)

small handful (80g) cooked peeled prawns

7 cooked king prawns
(I like the ones with a chilli dressing)

1 heaped tbsp (20g) prawn cocktail

80g freshly cooked crabmeat

80g can tuna, in water or brine, drained

½ 160g tuna in water or brine, drained

• Deli Ideas

6 large green olives

small handful (25g) small black olives

18 miniature marinated olives

4 baby char-grilled artichokes in oil, drained

75g char-grilled peppers in oil, drained

7 (40g) SunBlush tomato quarters, drained

1 wheat-free falafel (35g)

½ large hard-boiled egg

¼ small, ripe avocado

50g canned sweetcorn, drained

• Dips

2½tbsp reduced-fat houmous (25g)

2tbsp regular or flavoured houmous (20g)

4tbsp guacamole

8tbsp spicy tomato salsa

• Dressings and Sauces

½tbsp mayonnaise

1tbsp salad cream

2tsp *Body Blitz* dressing

½tbsp vinaigrette

1tbsp ready-made dressing

2tsp (10g) sunflower or olive oil spread

• Corn, Rye and Rice

2 rye crispbreads

2 rice or corn cakes

½ slice of rye bread with spread

2tbsp (15g) uncooked white rice

4 heaped tbsp cooked white rice

Snacks and Drinks

In the old days – before I discovered **The Rules** – I would eat very little most of the day and then pig out on bags of crisps, chocolate and sweets when I had an energy slump in the afternoon. If I felt unhappy, angry or frustrated, I would reach for the biscuit tin and stuff my face to take the pain away. The sad thing is, all these foods only made me feel worse, not better. And I knew it.

You need to weigh up which is more important – an unhealthy snack or the chance to finally and permanently lose weight. I've made my choice.

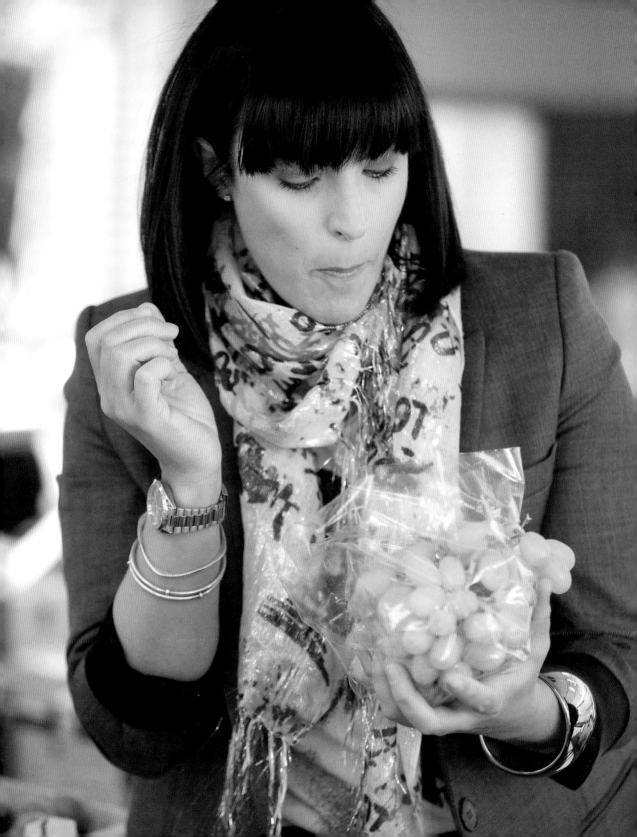

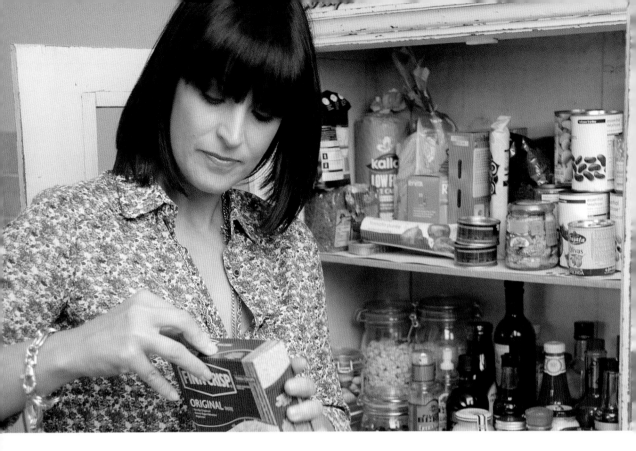

Corn Cakes and Rice Cakes

Yes, I know, eating rice cakes is like munching on polystyrene ceiling tiles. (Well, it is a bit.) But they are low calorie and make a great base for a variety of yummy toppings.

One large rice cake contains roughly a quarter of the calories of a slice of white bread. I know we're not really counting calories here, but as I've said before, they do make a difference. And as far as I'm concerned, any pain-free way I can cut the number I consume, the better.

Corn cakes are like rice cakes but made with – you guessed it – sweetcorn (maize). The ones I buy are thinner than rice cakes and have more flavour. I sometimes break them into chunky pieces to kid myself I'm eating tortilla chips.

Rye Crispbreads

Crispbreads are low in calories and fat, contain loads of fibre and can make a great snack – especially when served with toppings that taste much better than they do! They're particularly handy when you're following **The Rules** because they slot very easily into that 'I'm desperate for a snack!' time of day.

Although they take a bit of getting used to, I found that once I started eating them – a bit like rye bread – it wasn't long before I was looking forward to my mid-morning crispbread snack. So, get topping!

HERE ARE **10 QUICK TOPPINGS** THAT MAKE **10 GREAT SNACKS**. SERVE WITH UNLIMITED VEGGIES. TAKE 2 RICE CAKES, CORN CAKES OR RYE CRISPBREADS AND TOP WITH ANY OF THE FOLLOWING:

- 2tsp (10g) crunchy peanut butter
- Small handful prawns and 1tsp salad cream
- ½ thinly sliced banana
- 1tsp sunflower or olive oil spread, Marmite and sliced cucumber
- 1 heaped tbsp reduced-fat houmous
- 4 slices wafer-thin ham and 2tsp sandwich pickle
- 2tsp reduced-fat houmous, sliced tomato and 1 slice Parma ham
- 1tbsp guacamole and 2tsp spicy tomato salsa
- 2 slices roast chicken breast, 4 halved cherry tomatoes
- 2 sliced tomatoes and 2tsp salad cream

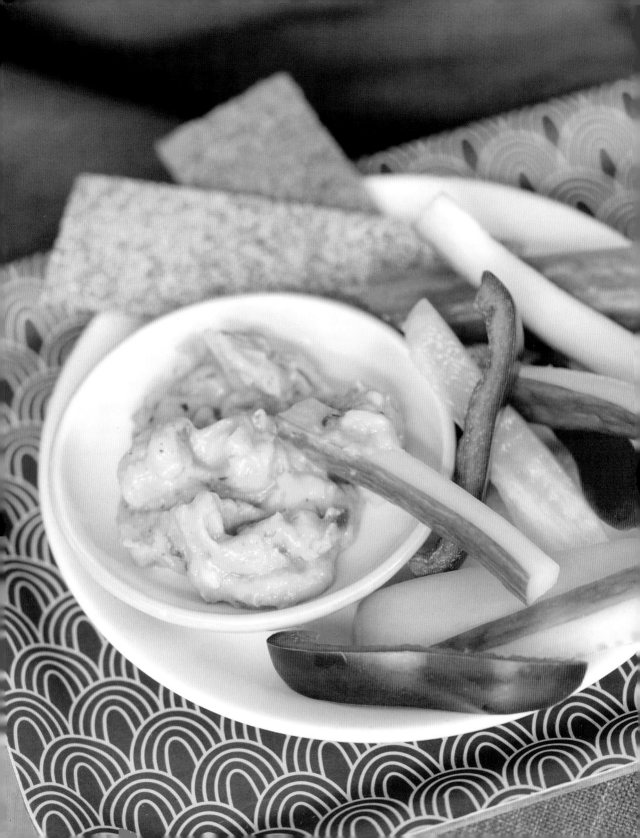

Dips

All supermarkets sell a wide range of dips and as long as you stay clear of the ones containing dairy products like cream cheese, yogurt and crème fraîche or those thickened with breadcrumbs, such as taramasalata, you can buy almost whatever you like.

Bear in mind though, most dips are blended with loads of oil to give them a creamy texture, so don't go over the top with your portion size. This is one occasion where it's OK to opt for the reduced-fat versions if you see them. (I also think that life's too short to bother making your own houmous. There are so many good ones in the supermarket, just make sure you buy the smallest pack you can, so you're not tempted to eat too much at one time.)

A couple of tablespoons of dip are plenty for a snack when served with heaps of crunchy vegetable sticks. And I do mean vegetable sticks. Do not use crisps, tortilla chips, Pringles, chipsticks or any other kinds of snacks for dipping.

Instead, prepare a load of vegetables such as carrots, cucumber, celery, peppers and cherry tomatoes. Keep in a plastic bag in the fridge ready to nibble when you have the urge.

Easy Dips To Make

These simple dips use lots of ingredients that you may have left over or knocking about in your cupboard and fridge.

• Roasted Red Pepper Dip

Drain a 290g jar of char-grilled roasted peppers and put in a food processor with 1 roughly chopped garlic clove. Add a pinch of salt and plenty of ground black pepper. Blitz until smooth. Use as a dip or a sauce for grilled chicken, meat or fish.

Makes 4 snack servings.

• Guacamole

Mash 1 ripe avocado with half a crushed garlic clove, a pinch of hot chilli powder and the juice of ½ a lime. Put in a small bowl and serve. (If there is any left over, you can cover the surface tightly with cling film and keep in the fridge for up to a day.)

Makes 3 snack servings.

• Houmous with Lime and Coriander

Mix half a 200g tub of reduced-fat houmous with the juice of ½ a lime, a pinch of ground coriander, 2tbsp of chopped fresh coriander and a few twists of ground black pepper. Serve with lots of vegetable sticks.

Makes 2 snack servings.

• Tapenade

Put 100g drained small black pitted olives, 1tbsp drained baby capers, 1 small roughly chopped garlic clove and a pinch of dried thyme in a food processor. Add a couple of anchovy fillets. Dribble over 3tbsp extra virgin olive oil and blend.

Makes 4 snack servings.

• Minted Broad Bean and Lemon Dip

Boil 200g frozen broad beans until tender. Rinse under running water until cold. Drain. Slip off all the skins and put the beans in a food processor. Add a small roughly chopped garlic clove and the finely grated zest of a lemon. Add 3tbsp of reduced-fat houmous and 2–3tbsp of cold water. Blend until smooth. Stir in chopped mint leaves. Add lemon juice to taste.

Makes 4 snack servings.

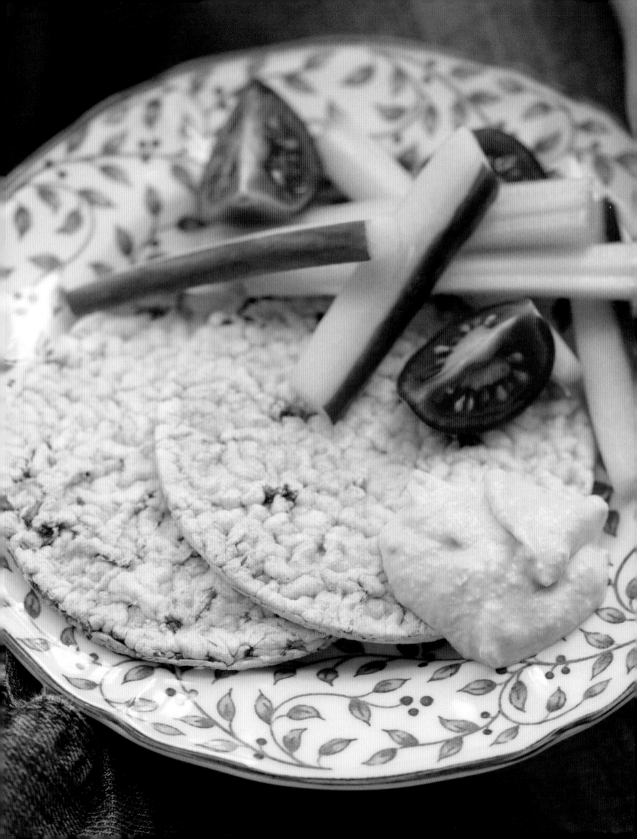

Nuts and Seeds

Nuts and seeds are hideously high in calories, but they're also packed with nutrients, essential oils and protein, so as long as you eat them in moderation you'll continue to lose weight.

I tend to buy fruit and nut mixes from the supermarket as the dried fruit satisfies my sweet tooth. I always keep some in my bag for snacking on whenever I'm tempted by something BAD.

Stay away from fruit and nut mixtures that have added sugar, honey or yogurt coatings. Those with cranberries, banana chips or coconut are particular culprits.

Dried fruit has an intense sweetness that can help curb sugar cravings, but don't eat too much. A handful of raisins or five dried apricots are enough for a serving.

The ideal portion of nuts for a snack would be just enough to fit into one cupped hand – no more than around 15g if you're measuring. If you are having a fruit and nut mix, you can have half as much again.

EACH OF THESE PORTIONS REPRESENTS **ONE** SNACK SERVING. CHOOSE UNSALTED NUTS WHERE POSSIBLE.

- 6 whole shelled Brazil nuts
- 8 smaller nuts like almonds or cashews
- small handful pumpkin seeds
- small handful sunflower seeds
- 2tbsp (15g) pine nuts
- small handful peanuts
- handful (25g) dried fruit and nuts
- small handful chopped mixed nuts

• Spicy Nuts

These hot and spicy nuts make a brilliant alternative to crisps with drinks.

Toss 100g plain mixed nuts with 2tsp dark soy sauce and ½tsp hot chilli powder. Scatter over a baking sheet and bake in a preheated oven at 200°C/Gas 6 for 5 minutes. Leave to cool before eating. **Makes 6 servings.**

• Homemade Popcorn

If you find it hard to stop nibbling in the evening, make a batch of popcorn and it should keep you out of the biscuit tin. You'll find plain popping corn in the natural food section of the supermarket. Keep clear of sweetened or salted varieties.

Mist the inside of a medium saucepan with mild cooking oil. Add a good handful (about 50g) popping corn and cover with a tight-fitting lid. Put over a medium heat and leave for 2–3 minutes. As soon as you hear the corn popping, give the pan a good shake. But don't open or hot popcorn could fly up into your face. Continue cooking until the corn stops popping, but make sure you shake pretty regularly so it doesn't burn on the bottom of the pan. When it's done, tip into a large bowl and leave to cool for a short while before eating. **Makes 2 servings.**

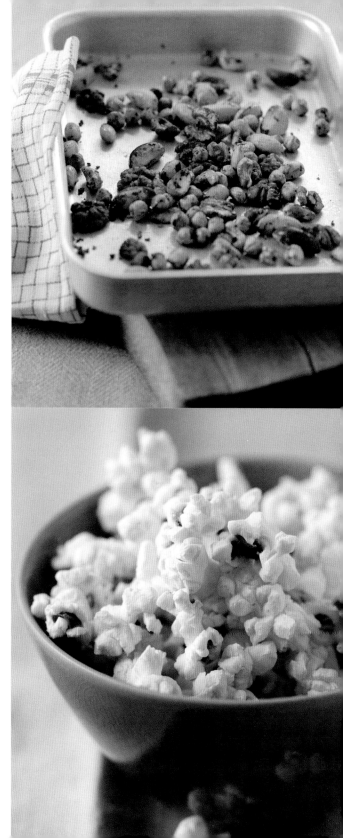

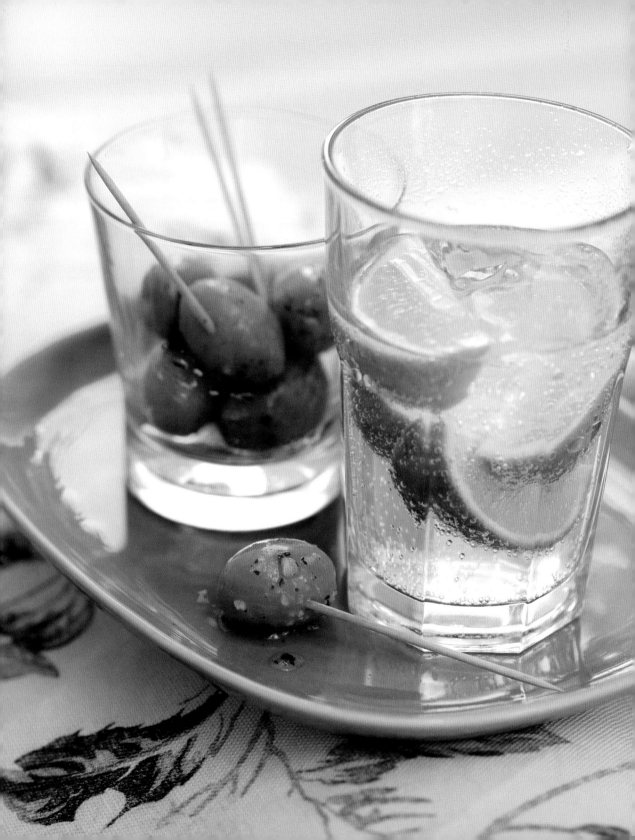

Drinks

Going without alcohol for two weeks can be a bit of a bind. But get over it! Treat yourself to one of these instead – at least you won't be waking up with a hangover.

Cheat's G&T

Half squeeze 2 lime wedges into a glass, add 3–4 cubes of ice and drop the lime wedges on top. Top up with well chilled low-calorie tonic.

Virgin Mary

Pour 250ml tomato juice into a glass and season with 1–2tsp Worcestershire sauce, a few drops of Tabasco, ground black pepper and a little salt to taste. (Use celery salt if you have it.) Add a couple of ice cubes. Stir with a celery stick if you have one handy, then nibble it while you sip your drink.
(Counts as ½ snack)

Lime Quencher

Pour 1–2tbsp lime cordial into a tall glass, add two wedges of fresh lime and a couple of ice cubes. Top up with well chilled sparkling water.

Ginger Zinger

Half squeeze 2 lime wedges into a glass, add 3–4 cubes of ice and drop the lime wedges on top. Top up with well chilled low-calorie ginger ale.

Elderflower Spritz

Pour 1–2tbsp elderflower cordial into a tall glass. Add 3–4 ice cubes, 4–5 thin slices of cucumber and a couple of sprigs of mint. Top up with well chilled sparkling water and serve.

Clementine Fizz

Squeeze the juice of 3 clementines. Pour into a glass and add a couple of ice cubes. Top up with well chilled low-calorie lemonade. (If you don't have any clementines, you can also use satsumas instead.)
(Counts as ½ snack)

Sparkling Orange

Pour 100ml fresh orange juice into a tall glass, add a couple of ice cubes and top up with well chilled sparkling water.
(Counts as ½ snack)

Cola Tang

Half squeeze 2 lemon wedges into a glass, add 3–4 cubes of ice and drop the lemon wedges on top. Top up with well chilled diet cola.

Real Life

I think one of the main reasons **THE RULES** have helped me succeed when every other diet has failed is because it's so easy.

Wherever I am and whatever I'm doing, I can eat loads of foods that obey **The Rules** and still lose weight. Any restaurant, café, supermarket, corner store or even garage forecourt sells foods that I can eat. OK, so sometimes it might be a bit more tricky, but there is absolutely no need to go hungry. A lot of people have told me that they worry about what they should order when they're eating out – simply because we can't control what gets put on our plate. Well now you can! It's time to take back the control...for good.

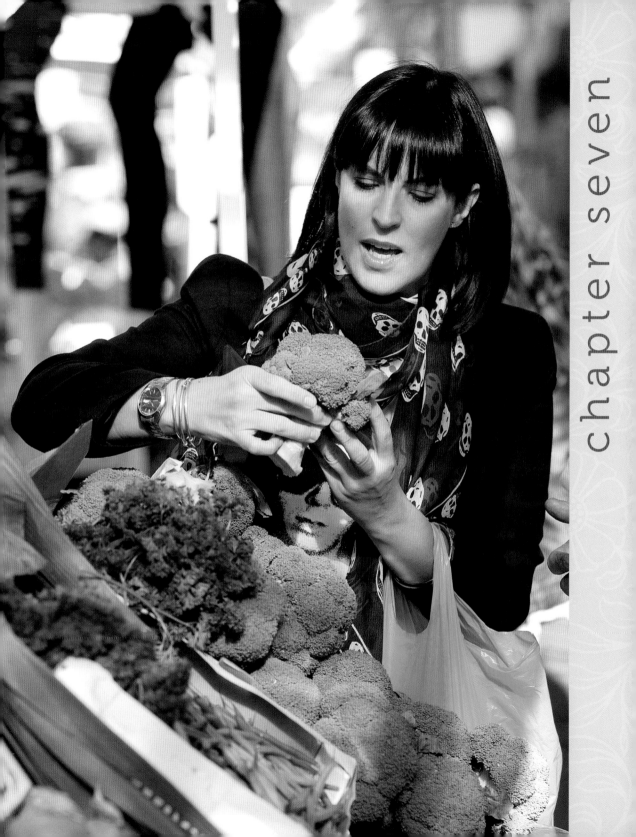

chapter seven

Eating Out

There are times when even with the best will in the world, you simply can't avoid eating out. But, don't panic. It is possible to follow **The Rules** and eat in almost any restaurant. Here are just some of the foods that you can eat out.

1. ITALIAN RESTAURANT

Italian restaurants and even pizza houses, like PIZZA EXPRESS, tend to be good places to eat because usually they offer a pretty wide selection of salads and grilled meats or fish. Make sure you keep away from the pasta, potatoes and any cheesy sauces though. And avoid the breadsticks like the plague as it's easy to mindlessly eat them. Always, always ask for the salad dressing on the side then you can control how much, if any, you want on your food.

Anna's Alternatives

- **Melon wrapped in Parma ham**
- **Selection of antipasti**
- **Tomato and basil soup**
- **Tuna and bean salad**
- **Grilled fish and vegetables**
- **Grilled meat, chicken or tuna and salad**

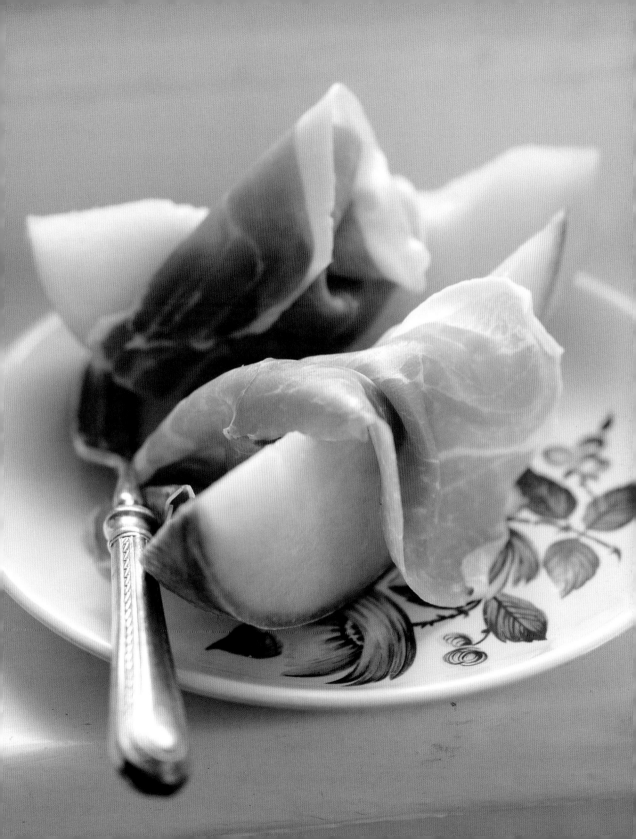

2. INDIAN RESTAURANT

It's even possible to have a curry, as long as it's not made with cream, yogurt or any other dairy product. Be a bit sensible though. Don't scoff your way through the whole serving. Just half is plenty for you at the moment, so share with a friend. Tandoori chicken and chicken tikka tend to be fairly low in fat, so would normally make a sensible choice. Unfortunately, they're marinated in yogurt, so you can't eat them for the moment. Save until the two weeks are up. Poppadums are made with chickpea flour, so should in theory be fine. But they're deep-fried in gallons of oil, so don't have them!

Anna's Alternatives

- **Chicken, lamb or prawn curry in a tomato or lentil sauce**
- **Dahl**
- **Rice dishes** *(lunchtime only)*
- **Tomato and onion salad**

3. CHINESE OR THAI RESTAURANT

Your local Chinese restaurant will probably offer a huge range of dishes, most of which are packed with salt, sugar and fat. If you must, try to choose the following. And no prawn crackers! They're greasy enough to use as lip balm.

Anna's Alternatives

- **Grilled chicken or prawn skewers**
- **Stir-fried chicken, prawns, vegetables and tofu**

- Rice dishes during the day – but not any kind of fried rice
- Dishes made with rice noodles in a simple broth or thin soup

4. LOCAL PUB

This can be problematic, but as long as you go for a salad or small portions of main meals, you should be fine. Ignore the bread and fill up on plenty of fizzy water from the bar. Limit yourself to just one sachet of dressing.

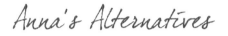

Anna's Alternatives

- **Vegetable soup**
- **Ham, chicken, beef, tuna, prawn, smoked salmon or egg salad**
- **Steak and salad**
- **Roast chicken or beef with a little gravy and lots of vegetables**
- **Chilli con carne and rice** *(lunchtime only)*

5. BURGER BAR

Ooh this is a really tricky one. But the best I can advise you is to go for a plain 100% beefburger and don't eat the bun. Obviously, anything with a crumb coating is out of the question, as are the fries. See if you can have some sort of salad with the burger. At the kebab shop, go for lean meat skewers, not the doner, and have lots of salad and no flatbread.

6. FISH AND CHIP SHOP

If you're going to a fish and chip shop you're on the wrong path
– keep away!

What Next?

So, you've reached the end of your 14 days following **THE RULES** and you should have dropped that elusive dress size and lost 7lbs, maybe a little more. Well done, that's brilliant!

After years of overeating, making the commitment to lose weight and sticking to a plan is a great achievement. Sometimes people lose a little less than 7lbs – perhaps 5–6lbs – but you should still congratulate yourself. It's more than likely that you've dropped a dress size even if the scales aren't registering the full 7lbs loss. However much you've lost, you should be slimmer, fitter and hopefully feeling rather chuffed with yourself. And rightly so.

But remember, changing eating habits takes a lifetime commitment. If you really want to lose weight and keep the weight off, this is only the beginning. So, please don't waste the past two weeks by relaxing too much now. If you return to your old eating habits, the weight will soon creep on again.

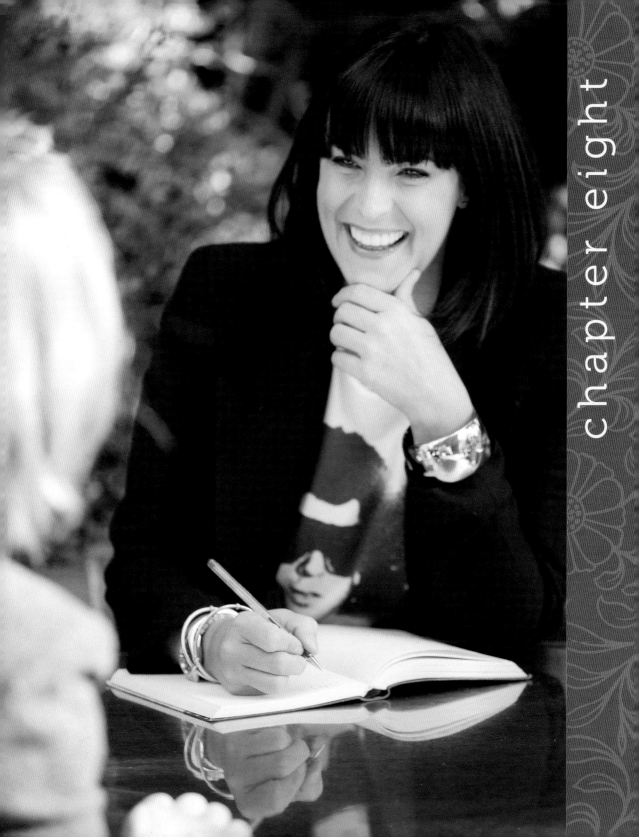

chapter eight

A Brand New You

Think about our *Body Blitz* plan as the start of a **Brand New You.** A new you destined for success not failure. If you only had a few pounds to lose you're probably well on your way to your target weight. A couple of stone or more and there's a little further to go until you reach a healthy, happy weight for you.

The last two weeks might have been a bit tough at times, but I have some simple ideas to help you through the next stages of weight loss. It's what's worked for me and what I've found suits my lifestyle. I'm not expecting you to never eat cheese or enjoy a glass of wine again. I think the occasional treat helps my weight loss because it stops me fixating on what I can't have and leads to a more natural way of eating.

So, now is the time to add some dairy foods, wheat and maybe occasional alcohol or treats back into your diet. I'd recommend sticking to the No Carbs after 6.00pm because it's a fuss-free way of helping you continue losing weight.

You can still use all the recipes and snacks in the book, or even follow the **14 Day Plan** again – but this time add small servings of potatoes, bread, pasta, cheese etc., keeping alcohol and treats for the weekend only. You should still be able to lose weight, but at a slightly lower rate – maybe 1–2lbs a week. It might not sound like much, but that's 7lbs a month. Do that for two months and you'll have lost a stone! Continue until you reach your ideal weight and you'll never look back!

Easy Does It

Be sensible though and keep away from massive portions. If you are following the **14 Day Plan** again, you can add three previously off-limits foods a day.

(They'll each need to contain around 100 calories.)

**FOR EXAMPLE, EACH DAY
YOU COULD ADD:**

- **1 small glass white wine**
- **1 small pot low-fat fruit yogurt**
- **3 small new potatoes**

OR

- **1 small baked potato**
- **1 thick slice white bread**
- **1 small piece of Cheddar**

For loads more ideas, check out my website
annarichardsonbodyblitz.com

For me, it's always the alcohol I miss most and knowing that I can sip the occasional glass of wine or a vodka & tonic at the weekend gives me something to look forward to. I also love potatoes, so incorporating them back into my diet means I can tuck into a baked potato. A little pasta with my Bolognese or a chunk of cheese now and then definitely helps keep me on the straight and getting narrower.

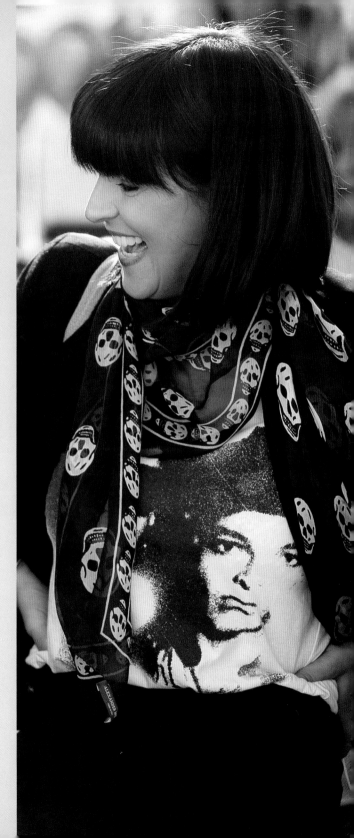

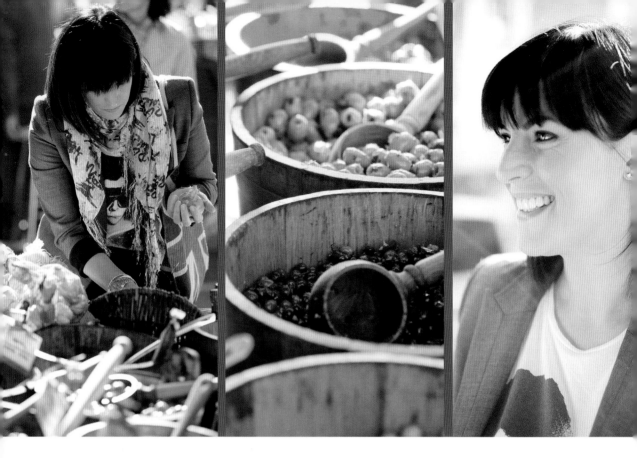

A Healthy Balance

It's especially important for women to have enough calcium in their diet. Two weeks almost dairy free aren't going to cause any health problems, but you shouldn't really be thinking about going dairy free for longer than a month or two without taking calcium supplements. Return some extra dairy products to your diet and you can stay pill free.

So, think about upping your milk to around 400ml a day and adding at least one more serving of calcium-rich food – a small pot of yogurt or a small portion of hard cheese. Or keep the milk the same and add two servings of calcium-rich food.

(If you're using soya or rice milk, make sure you buy the calcium-enriched versions.) Dairy products tend to be very high fat (and high fat means high calorie), so go for low-fat versions if you like, while trying to avoid those low-fat yogurts or desserts that are stuffed with sugar, sweeteners and stabilisers. Look at the labels closely. I also suggest you continue avoiding cream and keep the cheese down to a minimum for the moment. There will be times, no doubt, when it will be nigh impossible to deny yourself that dribble of cream on your strawberries, but keep those occasions few and far between and you'll continue to lose weight.

Treats

Talking to a lot of dieters, we've come across people who are addicted to chocolate and almost can't make it through the day without it. And those who love a biscuit at break time or a dessert after dinner. People who seem terrified by the prospect of cutting out sugary snacks for two weeks let alone for ever. So if this is all sounding rather familiar, fear not. Follow the plan for two weeks, lose the weight then perhaps keep the chocolate to weekends only – a bit like the alcohol.

Going Slow

If at some point your weight loss really slows down, if you haven't lost any more weight over a two-week period and you are certain that you haven't been eating too much or exercising too little, simply go back and follow **The Rules** for another 14 days. That should be enough to kick start the weight loss again. You should drop 4–5lbs, maybe more, depending on how much weight you need to lose overall.

Here's To You...

So I'm going to end where I started. With choice. Every day we make decisions that can help or hinder our health and happiness. Every day we're bombarded with temptation. And if you're a failed dieter like me, then it's just too easy to give in to the comfort of food simply because we're tired, emotional, bored or just addicted. Next thing you know, you're slobbing in front of the box with your backside bursting through the seam of your jeans pretending it doesn't matter.

I don't want to be like that. And neither do you. Which is why you've made the decision to change, once and for all.

So I'm going to raise a glass to you all and say 'Here's to you!' No matter how large or small your weight loss, you've made a big difference. To each and every one of us – **Well Done**.

If you'd like to stay in touch with Justine and me or simply find out more about my **Body Blitz** diet plan, we'd love to hear from you. Just log on to www.annarichardsonbodyblitz.com and we'll be waiting with a biscuit. Only joking.

anna xx

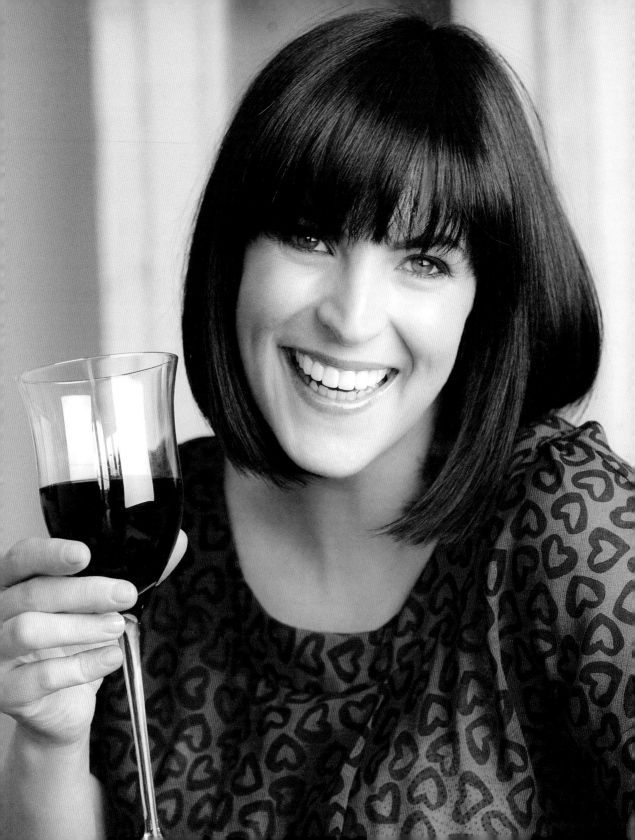

With Thanks...

From Anna...

It's such a small word and often gets forgotten. But 'thank you' can mean the world … I would never have been in such a privileged position to write a book had it not been for Channel 4. My love, respect and admiration goes to **Sue Murphy**, **Walter Iuzzolino** and **Colette Foster** for their genius minds and vision. Thank you. Where do I start with the hugely talented **Justine** and her team? Your passion and dedication to food has made this book a joy. **Jane** and **Lauren** – get back in that kitchen! I literally couldn't have done this without you and I know how very hard you've worked. Thank you. **Michael Foster** – one man, one agent, one legend. There's nothing else to say. I need to gather up all the thank yous in the world and post them to the publishing team at Orion, in particular **Lisa, Mark, Rabab, Gaby** and **Clare**. Very special thanks goes to my editor, the lovely **Amanda Harris** for your calm determination, laughter and addiction to cakes. A big thank you to **Nikki Dupin** and her design team. You had a mountain to climb – but you made it a beautiful Technicolor mountain covered in flowers, motifs, photos and fonts. Thank you. To the genius photographers **Karen Thomas** (www.karenthomasphotography.com), **Chris Gloag** (www.chrisgloag.com) and **Adam Lawrence** (www.adamlawrence.com). The pictures are good enough to eat. I've tried. Thank you! Thank you to **Jonathan Long** (no layers!) at **Lockonego Hair** (www.lockonego.com), make-up artist **Chloe Honore** and stylist **Kate Barlow** for washing me off, rinsing me out and scrubbing me up. Your task was not easy. A nod and a wink go to **Teresa Symes**, **Katie Walker** and **Michele Knight** – thank you girls. To **Mum, Dad OBE**, **Mark, Ben** & the family – aka The Munsters – thank you for being you. You are so very loved. A thousand kisses to the most talented **CM**. Your constant love and support is a blessing to me. Thank you. And finally, and finally… To My Friends and My Love. I sit in your shadow, always. Thank you xx

From Justine...

Anna, who would have thought that a morning arranging lobsters on your boobs and oysters in your navel would have brought us this far! Thanks for being such fun to work with and so damn committed to this book. **John**, who fancied me even when I was fat – although I know you prefer the new slim version. I will try to do more exercise in 2010. Promise. My two girls, **Jess** and **Emily**, for being great little cooks and trying everything. May you always have a sensible attitude towards food. **Mum**, for getting me in the habit of logging my weight daily – however bad the news. **Jane**, you're brilliant. Thank you for working incredibly hard and somehow always managing to keep a smile on your face. Well done for losing over a stone following **The Rules**! **Lauren**, for all the testing and your valuable input. I'm thrilled that working on this book inspired you to study nutrition at university. **Janet**, for keeping everything running smoothly. **Amanda**, for believing in the book right from the beginning. **Karen**, for your wonderful photographs. **Sarah Staines**, for sorting out all the legal bits and bobs. **Fiona**, for your nutritional advice and calorie calculations. **Lauren S** for your hard work and great ideas. All the wonderful women who gave their time to talk to us and share their dieting stories and secrets. Thank you girls!